THE RAINBOW PALACE

THE RAINBOW PALACE

TENZIN CHOEDRAK

With Gilles Van Grasdorff

Preface by the Dalai Lama

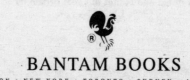

BANTAM BOOKS

LONDON · NEW YORK · TORONTO · SYDNEY · AUCKLAND

THE RAINBOW PALACE
Le Palais des Arcs-en-Ciel

A BANTAM BOOK : 0 553 81303 X

PRINTING HISTORY
Albin Michel edition published 1998
Bantam Books edition published 2000

1 3 5 7 9 10 8 6 4 2

Set in 11/13pt Palatino by Kestrel Data, Exeter, Devon.

Bantam Books are published by Transworld Publishers,
61–63 Uxbridge Road, London W5 5SA,
a division of The Random House Group Ltd,
in Australia by Random House Australia (Pty) Ltd,
20 Alfred Street, Milsons Point, Sydney, NSW 2061, Australia,
in New Zealand by Random House New Zealand Ltd,
18 Poland Road, Glenfield, Auckland 10, New Zealand,
and in South Africa by Random House (Pty) Ltd,
Endulini, 5a Jubilee Road, Parktown 2193, South Africa.

Printed and bound in Great Britain by
Clays Ltd, St Ives plc.

*To the Tibetan people,
to the Tibetan culture and medicine,
with a very special thought
for the monks of Chothey,
and for Men-Tsee-Khang.*

As long as there are suffering beings,
And until their illnesses are cured,
May I be their physician, their remedy, their servant.

Chantidéva,
'Initiation into the practice of
the Bodhisattva'
Chapter III, Strophe 8

Contents

Part Three: 1976–1998

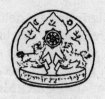

THE DALAI LAMA

Preface

I welcome the publication of Dr Tenzin Choedrak's autobiography. Dr Choedrak's story epitomizes the suffering of thousands of Tibetans over the last five decades. I hope this book will help create greater awareness of Tibet in the world.

Ironically, while in prison in Tibet, Dr Choedrak treated and cured many Chinese officials, winning the grudging admiration of his captors. The fact that hardened communist ideologues went to Dr Choedrak for treatment and cure – that, too, in the period when everything old and traditional was considered anathema – shows the efficacy of our medical system.

What is remarkable about Dr Choedrak, or many other Tibetans for that matter, is the fact that he harbours no feelings of hatred for his captors. All the time while he was being subjected to incredible hardship and torture, he did not lose faith in the Buddhist teachings that his tormentors were also human beings, having the seeds of Buddhahood, and like every one of us had fallen under delusion and adverse conditions. This belief saved the life and spirit of Dr Choedrak and many other Tibetans.

Since his arrival in India, Dr Choedrak has worked as my personal physician and Chief Medical Officer at the Tibetan Medical & Astrological Institute in Dharamsala, where many young Tibetans are being trained in the traditional Tibetan medical science.

I have no doubt that many readers of this book will be moved and inspired by his example of endurance and generosity. This book, I hope, will also encourage greater international support and concern for the plight of Tibet.

Tenzin Gyatso
Fourteenth Dalai Lama

Foreword

Knowledge of Tibet, its history, culture and religions is recent. Each piece of research that is carried out represents another stone in the construction of the edifice. This book is intended as a contribution to that process. Tibetology progresses with tentative steps, gradually bringing to light a country and a people threatened with extinction.

G.V.G.

Translator's Note

The Rainbow Palace was originally created from extensive tape-recorded interviews conducted by Gilles Van Grasdorff with Dr Tenzin Choedrak, in Tibetan. The tapes were transcribed into English and subsequently translated into French for the French edition of the book, *Le Palais des arcs-en-ciel* (Albin Michel, Paris, 1998). The present English translation is based on the French edition. Every effort has been made to use the accepted English spelling of the Tibetan words. The translator is especially indebted in this, and other technical matters pertaining to the text, to Jack Palmer-White, Paris, Tsering Tashi, Director, Tibet Center, Chicago, and Mary Alice Parsons, Chicago.

J.S.A.

In order not to interrupt the reader, footnotes and a glossary of names and words in common usage can be found at the end of the book.

Part One

1922–1950

1

Return to the Human World

My name is Tenzin Choedrak. By the Tibetan calendar, I was born the 15th day of the second month of the year dog-water. That would be April 1922. I was born to a poor family in a simple house in the heart of a country so old that it feels eternal. The mountains around us were majestic, covered with immaculate snow; the rocks were massive, and the vegetation was sparse. Our surroundings were rugged, but also rich with history.

My birth was premature. *Amala* [the familiar Tibetan name for 'mother'] had carried me only six months when I was born. On the day of my birth thunder rumbled so fiercely in the mountains that the villagers thought it might be the distant roaring of a dragon, provoked perhaps by my unexpected arrival.

The birth process is easily explained by reference to Tibetan medical texts. However, explaining the precise causes for a particular individual's birth is more complicated. Imagine the moment is at hand for your rebirth: you are in *bardo**, the intermediate state between

---

* Words followed by an asterisk the first time they appear in the text are explained in the Glossary.

15

life and death. Your spirit's need for a physical support grows more urgent. Impelled by karmic* energy, you approach your future parents at the moment of their sexual union.

Seeing them like that, you are seized by a strong emotion, you naturally experience a certain attraction for the one and aversion for the other. The *Gyushi** says:

Three substances are necessary to the formation of a body: first, a perfect sperm without defect from illness; second, menstrual blood [the Tibetan term for the ovum], which must be at the right moment of its cycle and also free of defect; and third, the spirit of the being in bardo *impelled by its karma. The five elements and their natures – earth, water, fire, air, and space – are also necessary to a being's physical existence. These are the conditions required for conception. Further development into male or female depends on the connections the being will make in its intermediate state. If it feels drawn to the mother and feels aversion for the father, it will be born male. On the other hand, if it is drawn to the father and feels anger toward the mother, a girl will be born.*

In my case I was born a boy. Was I meant to come back to pursue my spiritual path and help others? Only the human world permits this kind of progress. Toward the end of the pregnancy, the uterus becomes like a prison to the baby, full of revolting substances. In this dark fortress the baby feels intense sadness, repulsion, and uncleanliness. Only then does it prepare to leave its mother's abdomen. The moment of birth is a painful trauma for the infant. The *Gyushi* says, *The sensation of birth is similar to being skinned alive, or being stung by wasps, and when the infant is bathed, contact with the water gives the sensation of being struck.*

I do not know what I might have done in a previous life to be born prematurely. The explanation would be tied to my parents' actions and to the karma accumulated over the course of my earlier lives.

My family has always been very respectful of Tibetan customs and traditions. After *Amala* gave birth to me, she did not touch her hair or in fact any object. To do so too soon after my birth would be to risk losing whatever she touched. *Mola*, my grandmother (I prefer to use the Tibetan word for it is also an expression of respect), went to *Amala*'s bed and had her rub her hand over a small stone.[1] The third day[2] after my birth my family held the purification ceremony to free me of the birth impurities. It was still forbidden for anyone to visit the house because Tibetans believe the atmosphere inside the dwelling is still impure. Thus, it is necessary to wait until prayers and incense have done their work.

Amala washed her face and hair with warm water, put on clean clothes, and received the many villagers who came with presents to welcome me into this world. As Buddhists, we consider the human world the most precious of all worlds for it offers us the possibility of accumulating sufficient merits to reach Enlightenment.[3]

At dawn a month later a rainbow formed. There followed a black cloud, almost palpable, with twisting arms that imprisoned the distant monastery and then enveloped the hill closest to our house. And the rain fell, slanted and cold. Early in the afternoon a stocky black crow perched on a tree south-east of our house. At sunset it crowed mournfully and our dog barked six times. A few hours after these disturbing signs my mother, who was weakened by illness, left her physical form. My older brother was sixteen; I was scarcely a month old.

Many years have passed since my mother's death. Today I am a simple Buddhist monk. One thing I am sure of is that everything is impermanent.

The seventh Dalai Lama* said, 'Sometimes made up of happiness, sometimes misery, a human life is a fragile precious thing.' Though life be an apprenticeship, every being born on this earth must pass through the inevitable stages of birth, old age, illness and death. We have only to look around us to realize how obvious is impermanence. Nothing is stable, and it is equally true that nothing happens by chance. Every event flows from a preceding one. Even in our behavior we are not free. Our will and our desires depend on the sum of our past actions. We Buddhists call this the law of causality.

A person does not merely vanish into thin air at the moment of death. There will be a rebirth that may be happy, miserable, of a higher order or less good, depending on the dying person's state of mind and the quality of his or her karma. Most beings are powerless in the face of karma, which is why they must go through a rebirth. The maturity of the imprints left on the psychic continuum by past actions of body, word, and mind will shape the rebirth. This is why we ought to prepare ourselves long in advance of such prospects, as the poet Milarepa[4] invites us to do:

> *When you're strong and healthy,*
> *You don't think about the illness that may strike;*
> *But it hits you*
> *With the force of sudden lightning.*

Busy with worldly affairs,
You don't think about the approach of death;
Suddenly it surges up, like the storm
That bursts over your head.

Mola often told me about my mother's death. On that terrible night in the month of May the low hum of relatives, friends and monks could be heard tirelessly repeating the mantra of Chenrezik, the Buddha of Great Compassion, *Om Mani Padmi Hung**. Very early in the morning heavy gray clouds covered the mountain, and the thunder rolled louder and closer. At midday the sky cleared and bright colors splashed the countryside. Spirals of smoke from incense were still escaping from the altar when they draped my mother's body in a seated position in white linen. The lama said a final prayer with the family before carrying her to the nearby mountain, a mysterious place where vultures nest.

Mola told me that my father's pride would not let him express his pain, but that he sadly watched the lama until the man's outline merged with the horizon and seemed to be absorbed by a strange soft milky light. When the lama reached the consecrated spot, he set the body down as he intoned the prayers that penetrated the dense silence of the mountain heights. The sun's fire struck the earth. Way up high a sheet of snow, like a long stream of tears, suddenly broke away from the rocks, a farewell to the cherished being who had left this life.

The lama cut the body up, carefully detaching each shred of flesh, and threw the pieces to the greedy birds who had been watching; then he ground the bones, mixed in some *tsampa**, and left the mixture there. In

19

doing this, the lama made it possible for *Amala* to acquire a last merit as she crossed the stages of the *bardo*.

Today I am an old man. I do not know if I will live much longer: 'In the ocean of the Samsara*, our lives move like an eternally changing tide.' To escape from this ocean of suffering which carries us through birth, old age, sickness and death, we should tirelessly manifest goodness, love, compassion and equality of spirit toward all sentient beings. There is a proverb that says:

> *No matter where we live,*
> *If we are prisoners of the Samsara,*
> *We may as well dwell on the point of a needle,*
> *Which can bring no happiness or pleasure.*

It is unpleasant to remember a motherless childhood of many deprivations. But these were not my only sufferings. There is another period of my life of which the memory is painful. I refer to the twenty-one years I spent in prison, that marked me deeply. I remember with emotion meeting two old men from my village in a prison camp. I never saw them alive again. Most of those who shared our pain are no longer living, victims of the atrocities of the Chinese jailers. A few survived, like the monk Pelden Gyatso, who shared a cell with me for a year in the prison at Yititok near Lhasa. This memoir is intended to tell their story as well.

The past is heavy to bear. I could either consider it as over and done with and simply wipe it out of my mind, or I could meditate on the law of causality. Neither is easy. When memories assail me, I wonder if it would not have been better for me to withdraw from the world and become a simple hermit. Even today in Dharamsala[5], in the reception centers created by His Holiness the Dalai Lama, I am at every instant assailed with these memories. I am overcome especially with them when parents entrust their children to us to be given a liberal education so they may escape the Communist repression that still tries to crush our country.

Pala [the Tibetan word for 'father'] remarried a few months after my mother's death. My stepmother never loved me because I was not her son, and also I was considered to be the village simpleton because I had difficulty expressing myself. As a child, always dressed in tatters, I had no choice but to endure it all. My father was busy with his work, which often took him away from our home, and when he returned he had no time to listen to me. Anyway, as soon as he was back under the conjugal roof he had no authority. As for *Mola*, she had always known what went on in our home, but she had no say. I grew accustomed to suffering and finally no longer even complained about the bad treatment my stepmother inflicted on me. 'In the bed of the Samsara misery and shadows grow,' as the great fifth Dalai Lama said. I have never stopped meditating on this truth.

I must add that *Mola* loved me very much. She saw to me more than she did to her ten children, who were by this time older. While I was still only a newborn, she stole milk for me. In following years, since I was sleeping near her, there was not a single day that she did not secretly bring me a little bowl of fresh milk unbeknownst to my stepmother. Every evening before going to bed, she chanted her prayers and prostrated herself. I listened and watched her in silence, snuggled under a huge cover. She so much resembled the old women of the U-Tsang that you still encounter today in McLeod Ganj, upper Dharamsala. They are both rough and gentle, with love and compassion and serenity in their faces. When travelers took one of the three roads that led to the village and to our house, we always offered them a little swallow of *chang*, our barley-based beer. *Mola* dispensed the same hospitality to everyone, endlessly asking for news about Lhasa and Kundun*. Sometimes she told them stories about our family, mostly that the father of Kiabje Ling Rinpoche, the eldest tutor of His Holiness the Dalai Lama, and the *gyeltsap** of Tsourpou were related to us, but that we really had almost nothing to do with them. *Mola* unburdened herself tenderly over my fate, sharing with the visitors the secret of the milk she was stealing for me.

2

My Childhood as an Orphan

The name of my village is Niertchen. It is a two-day
trip from Lhasa, and almost as far from Chigatse.[6]
Long before my birth almost all the village people were
farmers with attachments to the Chothey monastery.
Niertchen was a beautiful place, but through the years
bad weather and poor harvests had impoverished the
people, forcing them to migrate. The only trace of their
presence was the ruins that surrounded my house and
where, as a child, I played with my friends.

Our house was at the foot of a hill, away from the
other dwellings. In summer, from the first rays of dawn
furtive shadows of praying people glided on the roofs,
their murmured incantations in counterpart to the jerky
movements of the prayer wheels. Incense would be
burning to attract the divinities' favors.

There were many tasks to be performed on our farm.
We grew barley, a little wheat, peas, and some mustard.
Fourteen people lived in the house: Uncle Tachi, Uncle
Tseten, papa Tetsen, Pasang, Poo, Dordje, Poutchoung,
Deki, Dreulkar, Nozom, my stepmother, *Pala*, *Mola*, and
me. My stepmother was the real head of the household
and she was stern.

When I was barely seven years old, not knowing what to do with me, she assigned me to guard our flock of seven hundred goats, sheep, and yaks. Every day at dawn I led them to the other side of the hill where a grassy plain stretched as far as you could see. We were all busy with our particular jobs. The work was difficult, the sun baked our skin, the tools scraped the dried earth. On evenings when the moon was full, we went back to work after prayers. Often, with the first rays of the sun, the older ones would already be at the water mill on the other side of the village preparing the *tsampa*. Their chants transported me and sitting on the top of the hill I would start to daydream. The gusts of wind whipped my face. I could hear the bleating of the flock grazing peacefuly nearby.

The fauna in Tibet was very rich. Musk deer, antelope, white-lipped deer and red deer would come up to the house. Bears, snow leopards and wolves kept an eye on our animals and came down from the mountains on stormy evenings. Ravens and crows also abounded. Sometimes I would catch sight of majestic eagles flying in the distance, and I tried to imitate them, turning in circles with my arms stretched out at my sides. But a shiver went through me as soon as a band of falcons interrupted their soaring to dive at a prey: death was on the prowl, and I ran to rejoin my nervous flock.

The flora was magnificent. An immense variety of wild plants grew on the side of the hill. Mushrooms formed a multicolored carpet; there were red ones and white ones, but the yellow were the tastiest. I enjoyed them right after they were picked, and we all especially appreciated when *Mola* slipped them into the fire. This mixture of grilled mushrooms and *tsampa* that I greedily sprinkled with a pinch of salt was a real feast. We would also find wild onions, a sort of radish that the children liked, and a plant that resembled garlic.[7]

Once the flock was in the pasture I would hurry to climb the hill. There I spent part of my time watching the stream which snaked along the side of the hill. Every morning I was joined by my half-brothers and sisters, who were my only playmates. We spent hours happily building reservoirs in the water for silvery fish that we caught in our hands. Their contortions amused us enormously. Our cries and laughter accompanied the magic instant when we opened the dam and the fish would be carried away by the current.

Another game consisted of building little temples like the ones we saw around us in the village. Having carefully selected stones and tiles, we raised the walls and positioned the roofs. The hill was scattered with these clumsy constructions, embellished with a prayer flag that *Mola* donated. When we had nothing, we rolled a little wool around a stick and planted it in the ground. We pretended to burn incense, all the while engaged in our minute work which took up entire days. We sang prayers whose words we did not know, but whose melodies floated in our memory.

On certain afternoons, when the sun struck the scraggly grass. I stretched out on the side of the hill and fell into a deep sleep, my head nestled against a kid. But when I was not able to find sleep, everything seemed confused. A single thought would then occupy my mind, that of my mother. Although I had not known her, I often had the impression of having seen her, though the image was scarcely perceptible. I took for a memory what was simply the fruit of my imagination, that is, the tender smile of my mother, *Amala*.

This presence helped me to bear my difference from my half-brothers and sisters. My stepmother was partial as far as we were concerned, giving the warmest clothes to her own children. I had a white woolen shirt that was full of holes and a torn *chupa** that I pieced together as best I could, and my shoes were worn down at the heel. I was so accustomed to this state of affairs that I became used to the cold that penetrated to my bones.

At nightfall I brought the flock back down home. The stables occupied the entire ground floor of our house. The hearth was located on the second floor, which we called the middle room. The top floor was reserved for the altar, the offerings, and the fireplace used for fumigating and purification.

The period of *Lossar*, the new year, is the occasion for multiple celebrations. In the monastery of Chothey, as in all the consecrated places in Tibet, the monks and the lamas conducted the *poudja*, the ritual offerings to the Dharmapalas, who are the protecting deities of the Dharma*. The new year is also the occasion for Tibetans to undertake a great house-cleaning. We sweep the house from top to bottom, repaint the walls and the altar; we change the prayer flags on the roofs of the houses and the monasteries – all of this in an atmosphere of joy. Throughout the month in every dwelling ceremonies of purification and collective prayers are held. We also exchange *katas**, the white silk scarf offered in place of flowers, and *khapse*, fried cakes, and we say *Tachi delek** to express our good wishes.

Men and women must cleanse themselves as well. On the day of *Lossar* Tibetans are obliged to wash their hair.

They dress in new clothes, or if they do not have the means for that, at least they put on clean ones. For *Lossar* as well as any other occasion of village festivities my stepmother's partiality was especially obvious: my half-brothers and sisters were all dressed in new clothes, but I continued to wear the same rags. I think that at the time many children without a mother lived this way.

In our house, as in the rest of the country, life would take on a contagious excitement. As soon as dawn broke, the altar was illuminated by little butter lamps which diffused a sparkling brightness. The haunting chant went up: *Om Mani Padmi Hung*. They say, and I really believe it is so, that this mantra is so engraved in the Tibetan memory that a child is capable of reciting it when he has scarcely pronounced the word *Amala*. Tirelessly the eldest of the family repeated the prayer to Tara[8], which the children murmured softly, pretending to know it already. Outside the prayer flags, which were part of the landscape, were tossed by the wind.

Every month our family received three or four monks, depending on our means of the moment. Tea was brought to them, meals served, and they were offered a little money. In return, during the reading of sacred texts they said prayers on our behalf. One thing amazed me during this period of my life: my family made much of the reading of the *Boumdrok* and the *Nyitri*[9], believing they were doing something exceptional. As I reflected on this later, I wondered why they were so proud of it. My stepmother would always say: 'I don't understand. In spite of everything we still get sick.' If they had thought about these words of the thirteenth Dalai Lama, my family doubtless would not have suffered so much.

The vain who cannot contain their happiness
Run here and there with childish excitement.
When they are sick, they weep loudly.
Unable to endure suffering,
They cannot live in contentment
Even for a moment.

This reminds me of the well-known story about the monk who lived in retreat in a grotto. One day, as he was waiting for the visit of the person who saw to his material needs, he decorated his altar prettily with bowls, offerings and butter lamps. When he had finished this arrangement, and as his benefactor approached, he realized that his motivation was not pure. He was trying to seduce his benefactor by creating the appearance of a pious practitioner. When he realized this, he threw dust on his altar and his offerings. A great master heard what had happened and declared, 'With their covering of dust, these were the finest offerings that could have been made in Tibet!' As a child I did not understand, but only later, when I had become a monk, did I understand that my family was not devoted to a true practice of religion. Because of this they accumulated vast quantities of negative karma, from which arose the serious problems they regularly encountered.

Let us consider the example of the Chinese, who have treated the Tibetans so badly. It is possible that in an earlier time we acted badly toward them. For my part, whether it was in the monastery, at home or in prison, I experienced very difficult, even tragic moments. However, many years ago I was the physician of his Holiness the Dalai Lama, and I became so again twenty years later. Life is a mixture of good and bad moments, of joy and sorrow, of happiness and profound pain. It can last a hundred years, but it is not our first life nor our last one. We pass through our lives in many forms before attaining Enlightenment. We have all been the mother, the father, the sister, the brother, the friend, the enemy of each living being.

So to purify our spirit, we must always seek to confront the consequences of the causes we set in motion. There is an edifying story on this subject. One day in the mountains, a mother was grinding a goat's head into powder that she then put into her *chupa*. Her child was tied to her back, and she regularly looked back at him lovingly. A starving dog arrived. The mother picked up the stone she had been using as a tool and struck the animal with it. A lama who was passing by observed this scene and went off smiling to himself. The reason for his reaction was that the woman had been carefully crushing the head of a goat which had been her father in a previous life; she had savagely struck the dog, who had been her mother; and she expressed the greatest tenderness for the child she carried on her back, although in a previous life it had been her worst enemy.

The story illustrates the advice of the Buddha to manifest a compassionate attitude toward all beings, for, at one time or another, every one of them has been our father or our mother.

The winter was harsh. The air was cold and damp, the streams froze over, and snow covered the land. Smoke rose from the chimneys in tight spirals. In spite of the discomforts, I loved this time of the year because *Pala* was there. Frequently in the wee hours of the morning I would join him in the stable. From there I would gaze out at the immense mountain chain. One particular morning was different from the others. I remember feeling at peace in my father's calm presence. A double rainbow rested on the next hill and suddenly a face that I knew had to be *Amala*'s appeared to me. She was smiling at me. What did my mother's presence in this place signify? I decided to talk to *Mola* about it. '*Amala* is watching over you,' she said. 'You know, Tenzin, the time has come for you to think about leaving our house. One day you will have to grow up without me. You can't stay here and be a servant to your family. In the monastery, you'll get an education and you'll have a peaceful life. Besides, your uncle will look after you.'

The decision was made: I would enter the monastery of Chothey at the end of winter. As we did every evening, the family gathered around the hearth. When *Mola* announced the news, the older family members did not smile, they just looked more solemn and continued to repeat *Om Mani Padmi Hung* and finger the *malas**, the beads we use for counting the repetitions. *Pala* had not uttered a word. He was in some other place, staring into the distance. He seemed so peaceful and also free. When he came back to us, he contemplated the fire for a little while longer; the blue and yellow flames flickering on the embers gave off a comforting warmth. Sitting close to each other, we watched *Pala*, who hugged me close to him. Then he began to tell one of the innumerable stories about Aku Tempa.

'Long ago when there were many local chieftains in Tibet, Aku Tempa was close to one of them and even became his secretary. This chieftain could not read or write but was a deeply devout Buddhist. In the beginning he was quite satisfied with Aku Tempa's work. But one day he became very irritated with him. The chieftain made him take off all his clothes which he then put on the roof of the palace. It was the coldest part of the year and, frozen to the bone, poor Aku Tempa shivered all night long. Early the next morning Aku Tempa on the sly took a little of the lime that was used for plastering the palace walls. He spread it carefully on the ground and did his business on it; then with a stick he traced some letters in his excrement. A few seconds later it was all frozen. Aku Tempa then stationed himself by an opening in the roof of the prayer room. He saw the chieftain seated cross-legged meditating before a magnificent altar dedicated to Buddha and all the deities. He waited for just the right moment and then dropped his work on the knees of the chieftain, who came out of his meditation with a start. Examining this strange object closely he saw the inscription. Since he could not read, he ordered his servants to fetch Aku Tempa but to serve him first a warm meal. A little later the chieftain asked him to read the "miraculous excrement". Aku Tempa respectfully bowed three times before humbly sitting down at the foot of the throne. He took the stick and read these words in a strong voice:

> *These excrements are from heaven;*
> *He who receives them on his knees*
> *Is the most fortunate of chieftains!*

Aku Tempa stood up and exclaimed: "Ah! You are the most fortunate of men to have them fall on you! You ought to eat a little to fully enjoy the benefits." The chieftain brought the strange mixture up to his nose, took a bite of it and placed the rest on the altar. Aku Tempa bowed deeply and backed out of the room.'

That evening the children listened more attentively than usual to this episode of the legendary tales of Aku Tempa told by my father. The older ones had completed their tasks. Toward midnight *Pala* took me to my bed. *Mola* offered me a bowl of *dri** milk, then made her prostrations. Sleep overtook me quickly. In a dream *Amala* appeared to me again and this time it was I who smiled at her.

3

First Steps to the Monastery

The winter of 1932 [the year monkey-water] was coming
to an end. In our village, there had been one birth and
two women had died. There was little illness in
Niertchen; the women were merely old and had come
to the end of life. Soon after my tenth birthday in April,
I led my flock onto the plain for the last time. The
light was harsh, the grass scraggly but growing and
scattered with wild flowers. This particular morning
it was especially cold and damp. It had been a long
time since my ragged clothes actually protected me.
They were so threadbare I could not even mend them
any more. As miserable and tired as I was, I heard
myself repeating in a low voice: *Om Mani Padme Hum*. I
became aware that my life was going to take place
elsewhere. One thing frightened me, however, and that
was having to leave *Mola*. Suddenly the light seemed
less beautiful. A feathery cloud crossed the sky just
above me. In a few moments many others appeared,
more dense, and gathered in the distance on the snowy
peaks. Soon it rained and the mud reached the hill
where I stood. But the mantra had its effect on me.
I felt serene and relaxed and experienced a sort of

excitement at the thought of leaving my family.

Down below the light was fading. I already sensed something important was going to happen. *Mola* had often said to me that at the Chothey monastery I would devote my life to love and compassion and to the protection of all life, human and animal. What she told me corresponds to the teachings of the Dharma which counsels us not to hurt others and as much as possible to be beneficent to all. Yes, this compassion that I would learn at Chothey I had already seen in *Mola*'s eyes and heard in her voice. This must also be a form of love.

Toward noon *Pala* joined me at the top of the hill. He caught his breath and sat down next to me on the riverbank. One of our dogs had followed him, and it jumped into my arms. I petted it tenderly. Suddenly it trembled, its ears went back, and it listened. I had also heard a strange noise, like a hissing. It was coming from a hole in the rocks where the wind whipped in, swirled and then brutally tore out again. The opening was larger than a terrier and concealed by bushes. The low noise grew more noticeable. The dog dashed inside, and a savage battle followed. A few seconds later it re-emerged with a snake in its mouth. All through my adolescence that sound, the wind, the wetness of the dead snake stayed with me as a picture of anguish.

For a long time *Pala* and I watched the village, which was emerging from winter and resuming its life. The days were warmer now, which allowed the villagers to see one another more often and renew their connections. The sun was low on the horizon, and a strange peacefulness settled around us. *Pala* announced our departure for the next morning. Within myself I felt calm, like being on a cloud or drinking a little too much *chang.* Before we left *Pala* gave me this advice: 'We let ourselves be led astray by the weight of our faults and illusions. But heed the profound and vast message of the Buddha:

> *Know that all things are thus:*
> *As a magician creates illusions*
> *Of horses and carts and cows,*
> *Nothing is as it appears.*[10]

Pala went back down to the house. Left alone, I felt the urge to murmur a prayer. It was inspired by the majesty of this place, the plain and the mountains blending into the horizon and seeming to hold many secrets. But, as usual, I did not have the words. Tears ran down my cheeks. I wanted to celebrate the surging of the dawn over the hill, *Mola*'s love and compassion, my mother's smile that I so often dreamed about, my departure for the monastery, the new life to unfold . . .

Clouds had encircled the hill. A first drop fell on the back of my hand with a resounding plop. I looked up to admire the slanted rays and stayed motionless watching the rain, soaked through. Finally I started down the hill. I let myself slide happily on the muddy ground and reached the bottom nose first in the icy water of the stream, which by now had become a small torrent. I arrived home in a sad state.

That evening *Pala* prayed to Tara to grant me the divinities' protection. Then *Mola* served the meal, which was *tsampa* dressed up with peas. A real feast!

In Tibet, it was considered a privilege to become a monk. For me, this was the beginning of a new life. Although she had nothing of her own, *Mola* took charge of my expenses, among which were the necessary donations to accompany my request for admission as well as the offering of tea to the monks of the monastery. She had also fashioned a little monastic robe for me. Pulling it on, I felt so proud and excited, as if I were going to celebrate *Lossar*, the new year. For the first time, *Mola* cried as she presented me with the *kata*. She solemnly advised me to apply myself to my studies: 'Become a good monk and always remember how uncertain life is and that circumstances can change as fast as a storm.'

In fact, Kelsang Gyatso, the seventh Dalai Lama, used to chant:

Life doesn't last, it's a setting sun.
Wealth, the dew on the mountain grass,
And the wind in the mountain passes like our praises,
Remember that a young body is a flower in autumn.

That morning seemed to me endless. They loaded up the donkeys with our things. *Pala* finally gave me the sign. A few more hugs and I could not contain my emotion when *Mola* pushed me toward the door. The road to the monastery was going to be long and unpredictable. In the dawning day, we climbed the hill on which I had nourished so many secrets. There was a last hesitation at the top, when I saw the altar I had put together the day before. I knelt down at it. My eyes blurred and I heard myself repeat: *Om Mani Padme Hum*. My father was already reaching the valley, which extended out of sight. I turned around toward our house and I saw *Mola* prostrate herself in our direction before disappearing into the stable.

At an altitude of about eighteen thousand feet and sometimes higher, we made our way slowly. The donkeys trotted a little ahead, followed by *Pala*. As I was not accustomed to walking such a distance, my body ached. By mid-morning we had crossed the valley. Then we entered a pass that led us into another valley. It was cold, the sky clear and the light even. Only tufts of grass grew here and there. Despite my difficulties in keeping up, my father did not slow the pace. I knew he was watching me out of the corner of his eye but he did not speak to me. He bent down to pick up twigs for the fire we would build at the next resting spot. I did the same but my arms were too short to carry them. We stopped at certain consecrated places where *Pala* applied himself to respecting the ancestral rites. He would sit down and pray. Prayer flags floated around us. The ground was strewn with *mani** stones placed by families to honor the divinities. Finally he unknotted our meager bundle that held the *tsampa* and the necessities for preparing the butter tea. Chants and nourishment gave me the serenity and strength needed for the ordeal. Then we set out again.

In the distance a dark mass in a lunar landscape finally appeared. A few monks moved about with extreme slowness, methodically, as if in a dream. We could make out a greener part where some children were running. I was fascinated but at the same time filled with anxiety, as if something were about to happen. It was, however, a pleasurable moment, serene and like a flowering.

We had walked for more than eight hours. Exhausted but relieved, we finally reached the monastery of Chothey, an immense building of at least five floors whose walls were the thickness of a man's foot. The first person we encountered was an old monk sitting cross-legged at the entrance. To protect himself from the sun he had covered the top of his head with a scrap of cloth, once yellow but now blackened by time. His face and body were emaciated. Motionless, only his lips moved weakly, and as he prayed his knotted hands fingered a *mala*. His eyes sparkled with a strange bright light. I thought I saw in them an expression of total goodness, of immense compassion, something I had always noticed in my *Mola*'s face.

My father led me directly to his brother Kelsang, my uncle and future tutor. In the monastery they almost never used the monks' given names; practically everyone went by a nickname. My uncle was called *Teu-ri-la* because he had a high round forehead.

After the customary presentations we went into a large hall in which there were thirty-two pillars. I especially remember my joy and emotion listening to the vigorous chanting of the monks as I watched the play of shadow and light produced by the butter lamps and discovered the statues of the Buddhas and the bodhisattvas*. My father made the offerings of the tea, white scarves, money, and *tsampa* mixed with dried fruits. My family's gifts were the occasion for several ceremonies and prayers to make my entry into the monastery official.

Pala gave me his final words of advice: obey your uncle-tutor, do not let yourself be distracted by the other monks. Then he disappeared into the shadows.

At that time the monasteries were the privileged places for the practice of religion. This was so for the four schools* of Tibetan Buddhism: *Nyingma, Kaguiu, Sakya,* and *Gueloug.* Attached to the principal monastery was a vast network of small monasteries spread out over the region. Certain sources indicate that Chothey, affiliated with one of the *Kaguiu* schools called *Bodong*[11], was built in the ninth century. A Chothey monk had become the abbot of *Guiuteu.* However, because a *Bodong* disciple cannot assume such a position, it is probable that some time earlier my monastery became affiliated with another school of Buddhism.

In the 1930s Chothey depended for support on about a dozen relatively wealthy families, *mi-ser,* and about forty small somewhat poor households, *doutchoung.* The wealthy ones shared the cultivated lands; the abbot conferred the menial work on the poorer families. When a *mi-ser* family came to own more than ten units of land, which could be of variable acreage, one unit was systematically donated to the monastery.

Every year around the eighth month of the Tibetan calendar there was a great celebration lasting for several days. Each family brought their part of the harvest. Tents were put up on the grounds of the monastery; there was praying and chanting, and the altar sagged under the offerings. It was the occasion for executing sacred masked dances and exhibiting innumerable butter sculptures, the detail of which could be amazing. The older people shared their own personal memories and also stories transmitted from their ancestors. They could spend hours conversing about the earth, weather, and harvests, all of it a subtle mixture of the sacred and profane. The discussions were lively and the divinities were frequently called on to protect the future harvests. Under certain special circumstances they would discuss events of the past, the legends of our region, the beginnings of our history.

Numerous ceremonies followed in succession. One especially was awaited by everyone with great anticipation. The family that had the best harvest was awarded the 'first place', and all of its members received a *kata*, the white scarf. On the other hand, the family that had presented the grain of the poorest quality got the 'last place' title. This explains why the families took such care with the lands and the harvest destined for the monastery.

The monasteries had their own code of conduct in the form of a charter, which clearly spelled out the rule the monks were to follow, whether or not you were a reincarnated lama, a *tulku*.[12] Anyone who disobeyed the rules, especially in the case of a serious transgression, had to leave the monastery. The rule of Chothey was very strict and dated from the reign of the Great Fifth Dalai Lama.[13] Everything here seemed to me so difficult, so inaccessible that I would silently plead for *Mola* to come to my aid. The first thing my uncle-tutor taught me was how to sit for prayers in the lotus position, like a rock pierced through by a sword, spinal column straight, eyes focused on the end of the nose. In the temple the slightest movement put you at the risk of the discipline master's whip or my uncle-tutor's nimble hand. There is a proverb that goes:

> *Don't fear the gods,*
> *Don't fear the phantoms,*
> *Fear only your tutors*
> *When they prostrate themselves.*

This means that when the dicipline master humbles himself in such a way he is preparing himself psychologically to administer a correction to his pupil. The act of prostration helps him to master his pride.

The day began at sunrise when the monks gathered in the great hall of the temple. Each day the program was full, often painful. There was the recitation of mantras and soutras (the Scriptures that carry the original teachings of the Buddha). Tantric meditations followed according to the days and the study sessions. Around eight o'clock in the morning we were served tea, then each of us joined his respective tutor. The primary task was to eliminate in each of us negative tendencies, such as attachment, anger, ignorance or laziness, which could sometimes get the better of novices and monks. But the exercises were also intended to guide us to an expansion of the spirit, to teach us love, compassion, and self-discipline. They changed with the hours of the day and ended around six o'clock in the evening. The adult monks would have dinner and then return to their work, while we novices would go to bed after another hour of reciting everything we had studied during the day.

The next day after the chanting and the morning meal I would go to my uncle Kelsang. I was expected to learn the texts by heart. This was a true ordeal. At the start of my novitiate I was regarded here, too, as a simpleton, so much difficulty did I have assimilating some of the teachings, which seemed nebulous to me. According to Buddhist principles, it is the tutor's obligation to criticize and scold but also when necessary to strike his pupil. My uncle did not hold back. If during the very first weeks of my monastic life he was somewhat understanding, he soon let me see how demanding he really was. At Chothey, they called him 'The Chinaman'.

But as I reflect on it now, my uncle's attitude was entirely appropriate. The more the tutor establishes a close relationship with his student, the better he knows and understands him and doubtless the more he feels the need to incite him to progress. As soon as something was not right, in proportion to the seriousness of my failings he would correct me and with whatever was handy, a whip, a switch, a stick. I was especially fearful of the alphabet classes. In the evening when I was tired and having trouble falling asleep, my thoughts would fly to *Mola* and, for an instant, the desire to flee the monastery would come over me. But I knew that if I actually did run away, I would bring shame on my family. So, in the monastery, too, I resigned myself to my fate.

I had become a fearful child. But I would look forward to the hour designated to go to one particular professor, a man of great goodness who never raised his hand to anyone. All the other novices shared my feeling for him.

In the afternoon the apprenticeship in calligraphy was for me another ordeal. The traditional method used to learn to write the Tibetan language consisted of transcribing letters on a birch or walnut plank that served as a blackboard. One side was painted black and varnished. The student would first cover the surface with a white powder and then, armed with a bamboo stylus, would painstakingly trace the letters following the method indicated by the master. When the blackboard was entirely covered with letters, the student would clean it and the operation would start all over again. Here in Chothey, however, the method was different. The masters gave us sheets of paper on which letters were written, and we had to read them over and over until we had memorized them.

Certain afternoons were given over to tasks. Excrement from horses, yak and sheep was used for fuel and manure; the novices had to collect it and spread it on the cultivated lands. And if other tasks came up, we had to tend to them without delay. We had scarcely a moment for relaxation, except when our professors were called away, usually to ceremonies that we novices did not attend. We made the most of such respites.

The *tsampa* rations frequently were insufficient and we were almost always hungry. When we were working in the fields, we would sometimes pocket a few potatoes on the sly. My uncle-tutor had a fireplace, so we would watch impatiently for the moment of his departure and then roast our potatoes on the glowing embers of the hearth. After this feast, we would hurriedly clean the place up and throw the cinders into a ditch.

Sometimes our tutors slept in the monastery kitchen. At midnight on such nights if the sky was clear, several of us took advantage of the magical moment when silence reigned over Chothey. We walked on the path that ran around the temple, with little steps, stooped over, to imitate our elders. Hugging the ground, we were furtive shadows that glided, knelt, arose and glided on. It was a moment when I felt physical pain leave my body and I became light, oh so light. Thanks to the murmurs, prayers and prostrations, I was happy.

Often our professors took part in prayers from which we were excused. We did not waste a second tearing along the paths of the monastery and off to a narrow canal that crossed through a park. It took us no time to throw off our monastic clothes and jump into the icy water where we swam naked. We would also build little irrigation canals and we designed roads that led to an imaginary windmill. Our laughter was loud and merry.

When I was twelve years old, I had a strange dream that I promised myself I would make come true as soon as possible. I confided my secret to three other novices. That started us off concocting wild plans to imitate the exploits of our elders who had made the pilgrimage around Mount Kalaish, that famous mountain that was an object of veneration for Tibetans. And after Mount Kalaish, why could we not go to India, to Bodh-Gaya where the Chakymouni Buddha received enlightenment?

We had no idea where India was, even less Mount Kalaish. We imagined sublime landscapes where an endless horizon blended into vast desert expanses. We made up our minds soon after *Lossar*, the new year. Our plan was simple, bold and completely crazy. We prepared a spartan bundle, a little *tsampa*, a few potatoes, and each of us packed one warm garment. We questioned the old monks carefully to determine which would be the best route to follow. So as not to arouse the least suspicion, we asked general questions about the region. The monks just took us for inquisitive novices and laughed at us.

The departure day arrived in spring. We had tried to conceal our nervousness. After the evening prayers we returned to our dormitory and waited for the monastery to settle down for the night. With a heavy heart I asked myself if this were a sensible thing to do, but there was no question of turning back. To build up our courage, we recited some mantras before blowing out the petrol lamp. Seconds seemed to last an eternity. Finally, I slipped out of my bed, followed by my three companions. We took our clothes, rolled up into small bundles, and went out with infinite precautions.

We had chosen this day for a simple reason: the full moon would help us follow our path until daybreak. Outside, the night was clear and cold. Quickly we put on our robes. By the position of the moon I calculated that it must be about two o'clock.

After we had gone through the first mountain pass, we noticed dark shadows of yaks against the snow. We made our way slowly. At daybreak fatigue overcame us and we had to stake out a spot where we could conceal ourselves. On the edge of the path there were small structures that sheltered relics, statues of Buddha and *mani* stones. These places were considered sacred, normally no-one went into them. But our legs would not carry us further, and we absolutely needed to sleep. Protected by the local deities we fell asleep, pressed against each other.

We were awakened by the howling of wolves in the distance. We shared the *tsampa* and the two remaining potatoes. As we were about to start out again, we got into a heated discussion. One of the boys refused to go on with this crazy adventure and urged us to turn around and head back to Chothey, which he did, alone. But once back at the monastery, he informed our tutor, who had no trouble finding us. Our return was swift and we received reprimands and corporal punishment. That night in my bed, however, I promised myself that one day I would go to Bodh-Gaya and Mount Kalaish.

*   *   *

Scarcely two years had gone by since I entered the monastery. In the eighth month of the year dog-wood [1934], I returned to visit my family for the first time. Before leaving the monastery, I took part with the other novices in some festivities that lasted a week. The meals we were served were delicious. The last day after a final communal ceremony our tutors gave us our freedom for a whole month.

That first year I especially appreciated the family reunion. It made me forget my uncle-tutor and the harshness of life at Chothey. At home everything was going on as before. I led the flock into the valley on the other side of the hill. But as soon as I had a little free time, I would find *Mola*, and we would have long talks. For a few days I resumed my old habits of sitting at the top of the hill and building little altars, all the while murmuring prayers. The only difference with the past was that now I knew the meaning of the mantra *Om Mani Padme Hum*. And all my thoughts remained fixed on my mother, *Amala*, in the beyond.

4

A Young Monk at the Monastery of Chothey

After I turned thirteen, studying texts became easier. I
had the feeling that reading them and the pleasure
I derived were enough in themselves. Certainly I did
not grasp all the meanings, and I still was not making
a perfect connection between the letter and the spirit.
Like many other novices, I was certain that it was
enough to possess a firm conviction to put the Dharma
into practice, an error that I later understood. Let us
suppose that the maximum length of human life is
eighty years. For the first ten years it is not possible
to realize the Dharma; and during the last twenty
years, we are less and less capable because of our
advanced age. During the fifty-year intermediate period
of life, the nights are for sleeping and the days for
working at our labor, fighting our enemies, and watching over our loved ones. In the course of a life it is
in fact difficult to find adequate time to study the
Dharma. We should also never forget that life is fraught
with uncertainty and that our determination must be
firm to live in accordance with the Law of the Buddha
and the teachings of the spiritual masters. That is
why it is essential to arrive at an understanding of

the 'law of karma', which concerns the cause-and-effect relationship between an action and the result that it produces.

The conviction regarding the Dharma became especially clear to me in my solitary encounters in the temple with the numerous representations of the deities. If their presence troubled me, they also gave me strength. I had a different approach to the texts when, a little later, I followed dialectical teachings. I really believe the sacred writings cannot be truly understood if one has not participated in these debates of logic. It is true, the practice of the Dharma is not an easy thing. The more one studies it, the more one becomes aware of its principles.

Like everyone, I sometimes get irritated, but the main cause of our sufferings proceeds from our actions. I spent long years in the work camps. I could hold that against the Chinese, but what would be the point? Our sufferings are born from an undisciplined mind, and this comes above all from ignorance. It is therefore necessary to control the mind by stopping the current of negative thinking. By persevering and concentrating on the body's physical reality, which is impermanence, and on the mind's psychological structure, it is possible to succeed in transforming this flow and calming the mind's agitation. We are all capable of applying ourselves to personal development, even to realizing *jampa* [goodness], *nyingdje* [compassion] and *cherap* [wisdom]. Comprehension of the ultimate nature, that is, of the phenomena that characterize vacuity, is the goal of one aspect of wisdom.

A Tibetan proverb says:

When the sun takes reasonably good care of a monk's needs
for clothing and nourishment,
He sets to practicing the Dharma.
But if he falls on adverse circumstances,
He becomes an ordinary man.

This means that it is easier to behave honorably when life's circumstances are favorable. While under constraints or in untoward conditions, the individual's reactions are more unpredictable. I met many men and women in the Chinese prisons: lay people, monks, *gueshe**, lamas. Many of them were good people. However, some also resorted to slaughtering pigs, beating and torturing prisoners in the service of our jailers. One of them was called Jampel, but I can cite numerous names. Many Tibetans succumbed under their blows. The venerable lama Bodong Tchokle Namguiel used to repeat: 'No individual can really appreciate the character of another.' I find this remark most pertinent. People who might look ferocious can prove to be good, generous, and courageous in suffering; others, pleasant and kind at the start, can turn out to be bad from self-interest as much as from weakness. We should never trust appearances or draw hasty conclusions from them. During my first two years of monastic life, my uncle was so strict with me that several times I almost ran away. But I learned never to judge him or hold it against him. It was with him that for the first time I experienced patience by trying to repress my revolt and not lose my temper.

That was not always easy. Daily life could be quite harsh at Chothey; the novices sometimes forgot the Dharma, especially when it came to playing a mean trick on a little schoolmate. They may have thought of me less and less as the idiot of the monastery, but I was still often singled out as a victim. This was most likely to happen in the spring, the time of the year when snakes slithered in the garden. Since my earliest childhood, I had a visceral fear of them. My schoolmates knew this and took advantage of it. I remember the day in particular when a young monk had received a visit from his family.

'*Amala* made barley cakes. I know you love them. Take one, Tenzin, it's for you . . .'

Carried away by my greediness, I plunged my hand into the sack.

I felt something viscous between my fingers and this thing began to entwine itself around my wrist. Instantly I understood that it was a snake and, terrorized, howling, I dropped the sack and the cakes and ran as fast as I could. It took me a long time to calm down, but once my fright had passed, I decided in the future to fight it out with kicks and punches. After the first scuffle, we were careful about where we fought, because we realized a monk was always around and punishment would be immediate. I worked hard at my studies, so when I was caught and punished for fighting, I felt frustrated.

As a young novice, I watched with envy the monks who paid visits to families to perform rituals and prayers. My turn came to go with them. This was an important moment in the monastic life of novices. We would be given a little money, much better and more substantial meals than at the monastery, and for a few hours escaped from our professors' surveillance. The families in the area asked for me more and more often to recite *chapten*, prayers for a long life, because I carried out the rituals faster than the other monks. These requests brought me great happiness. Then I remembered this story about Aku Tempa, told on a winter evening by *Pala*, my father.

Aku Tempa was a brilliant reader. Families often invited him to read in order to assure themselves of good fortune and prosperity. One day he was invited by a family to pray for several days. The father was completely bald. Because of this embarrassment he refused to participate in any public event, preferring to stay cloistered at home. When he absolutely had to go out, he wore a special head-covering that concealed his baldness. The days passed. Aku Tempa said the prayers in a confident voice. Tradition required that especially fine meals be served to readers, but they gave Aku Tempa only green beans and never any meat. He was distressed by this, but had an idea about how to remedy the situation.

This family owned a large flock of sheep, some black and some white. The father did not know how to read or write and of the sacred texts he knew only what people told him. At daybreak on the third day, Aku Tempa resumed his reading and, raising his voice, made up his own prayer:

If he who has not a single hair on his pate
Wore on his head the still-warm skin of a black sheep,
He would see his hair grow again!

Hearing these words, the father suddenly sat up straight.

'Is it true what you said?'

'Certainly,' Aku Tempa responded. 'They are the Buddha's words!'

The poor man believed him and sent a member of his family to kill a black sheep. He grabbed the still-warm bloody skin and put it on his head. That day Aku Tempa was served mutton for both lunch and dinner.

A few days later the poor fellow was still wearing his strange headpiece. The skin was beginning to give off a strong odor of decay. Aku Tempa had to invent a new prayer:

> He who wears the skin of a back sheep
> longer than a day
> will never see a hair grow on his head.

'What?' the man shouted. 'Read that again!'

Aku Tempa reread the prayer and explained: 'The Lord Buddha says that he who wears the skin more than a day will not see his hair grow back. Since you have had it on your head for several days, it is obvious you will never have any hair!'

The man was most unhappy and threw away the skin. Aku Tempa continued his reading.

Time passed. One day my tutor offered me an image of the thirteenth Dalai Lama, who had recently died in 1933, the year bird-water. It was in very bad condition but became one of the most precious treasures of my life. It took me a good week to fashion an amulet for it with a piece of silver that *Mola* had given me. Once finished, I proudly hung the image around my neck. Until then I had not seen a picture of Gyalwa Rinpoche[14] – another name that we give to the Dalai Lama. At home we had only small statues of Chenrezik and Amitabha[15].

At this time, I had become aware of the importance of my monastery, birthplace of Lotchen Bero, a great scholar of Tibetan Buddhism. I especially enjoyed the rare moments of solitude in the temple. From my thirteenth year I loved to hear the elders talk about the history of our monastery. Their stories sometimes transported us back entire centuries. In the ninth century King Langdarma[16] carried out a policy that was extremely hostile to Buddhists. He ferociously persecuted monks and lay people. His hirelings destroyed whatever concerned the Buddhist religion, killing monks, sacking and demolishing buildings, books, relics, everything.

Numerous statues were mutilated with nails driven into the feet and hands of the Buddhas and the other deities, and limbs were torn off. In certain monasteries, ours among them, I was told there were miraculous signs, such as statues that began to speak. It is thanks to these miracles that Chothey was saved from destruction, while two religious buildings, Sangri and Tak-Chouk, and a fortress, Dessi Rinetchen Dzong, a few kilometers from there, were totally razed. Only a few monks were able to flee the massacres and reach Chothey. They had brought with them quantities of sacred works. One of the most precious was composed of thirty volumes of four hundred and fifty to five hundred pages of text, each volume conserved between two planks of wood engraved with effigies of Buddha enhanced by gold. There was also a collection of sixteen *thangkas**, paintings on silk based on the sacred art, and innumerable statues and relics. As a result, Chothey became one of the most venerated places.

When I went into these sanctuaries, I would be overwhelmed by a profound emotion. From then on I became aware that complex things were by nature unstable, that human life was impermanent. I also loved moments of reflection and prayer at daybreak, that instant when, just before diappearing, the stars become almost imperceptible. The blackness lightened little by little, and I would be filled with awe. Sometimes a storm broke out over Chothey. Then the stars that had become invisible entered my heart. *Amala*, my mother, was smiling at me. Often I had an impression of seeing her image; in fact she had never left me. The monotonous course of my life was suspended when my feet took me wandering in the different rooms of the monastery. As I moved through them, I had only to close my eyes for images to surge up that are still with me today. The moments that I was happy in this life were rare. But in Chothey I was content, especially when everything around me became peaceful and conducive to meditation.

A statue of the Shakyamuni Buddha[17], the height of a two-story building, occupied the center of the principal hall on the ground floor. At his side were statues of Chenrezig and Tsepakme, the Buddhas of longevity. All three were in bronze and plated with the finest gold, giving the sanctuary a feeling of tranquil force. In this same hall I often stopped, thoughtful and sad, before works that had suffered mutilation or pillage. On leaving, I remained a moment in a slightly smaller room, which held a statue of the great erudite Bodong Tchokle Namguiel. Here the walls were covered with a paint with a gold base. On the first floor there were only two rooms. In the first one, reserved for prayer, they conserved the *Kanguiour*, which was more than a hundred manuscript volumes and about a hundred others composed of engravings. In the next room were kept thirty volumes of soutras* and a stoupa, which in symbolic fashion is the structure representing the body of Buddha. This particular one contained relics of a holy lama, Guedune Lhundroup, whose body had been preserved in salt. They told me later that when the Chinese laid siege to Chothey in 1950 and destroyed this stoupa, you could see hairs growing on the mummy's head. It is also here that the statues of the neighboring monasteries were reinstalled, lined up in staircase fashion. Some were the height of a man. Of inestimable value, they were all made entirely of metal, alloys of gold, silver, bronze. There were also paintings and the *thangkas*[18]. Finally, the third floor consisted of a single room that we called *Kaptchi*. There you could find the hundred or so volumes of the *Kanguiour*, also engraved on wooden blocks, and thirty volumes of commentary of Bodong Tchokle Namguiel printed on a thick rice paper by means of an ink composed of gold and silver powder. Numerous writings were conserved there as well as relics and statuettes of Buddhas and bodhisattvas. The texts, wrapped in squares of cloth or silk called *Ga*, were arranged between two planks of wood that bore engravings of divinities. These were then fastened in such a way as to keep the rice paper perfectly flat. On this same floor a last sanctuary held the stoupa of a great Tibetan scholar, Pang Lotsawa or Pang-Lo-Tchenpo. The statue of a divinity of the region, Tachi Ouanpak[19], and other effigies filled this place to protect the relic. Cushions and folded blankets were scattered on the floor to permit the monks to sit and meditate. There were also cymbals and other religious objects used in ceremonies. The third floor also held very old statues which had belonged to Chothey since its founding. The rest of the building was used as lodgings for the monks and guest rooms for passing travelers and pilgrims.

Most of the Tibetan monasteries were built on the top of hills, but Chothey was situated on the side of a deep gorge, crossed by a river whose roaring waters especially attracted me on fine days. A suspension bridge made of wooden slats and bound by cables and ropes permitted people to cross. However, pack animals could not pass over it. One side of the monastery looked out on the river, and the other sides overlooked gardens. Here is where the dormitories of most of the monks were located. A narrow path, which I took every day, ran around the building.

I especially liked the second floor of the principal building, because there were vast open spaces which looked toward the north onto the garden. With my legs dangling, I would sit alone on the low stone wall. The strong wind penetrated the openings with high-pitched singing. I felt transported and when my hearing became accustomed to the environment, I listened attentively to the rustling of the trees, which threw their shadows below. This garden welcomed numerous coucous and other songbirds, one with a red beak and black feathers that we call *jeumo*. I was also fond of this marvelous place for its little pond where, it was said, Lotchen Bero used to bathe and for its poplar which would burn with bright colors in the autumn. Sometimes I brought texts with me and studied there while eagles soared over my head. I knew they saw me from a distance, and I told myself that *Amala* and *Mola* were present in this setting that was inscribed forever in my mind.

In 1938, the year tiger-earth began like all years of the Tibetan calendar with ceremonies celebrating *Lossar*, the new year. This year I turned sixteen and it was to prove to be a year quite different from the others. In fact, I had decided to become a doctor – in Tibetan, *amchi*[20]. Circumstances now were going to help me attain my goal.

This decision was henceforth buried in the deepest part of me. The preceding year I had rejoined my family for the vacation period. One day an amazing man arrived at the house. He proudly wore a beautiful yellow brocade shirt. *Mola* had received him by lighting incense, which was generally done in the presence of lamas, important *tulkus** or great savants. She also served him tea and a delicious meal. Intrigued by his learning, I questioned him. He told me that he had followed long years of study at Chagpori[21], the medical college of Lhasa. 'Yes,' I thought, 'I will be an *amchi*, too.' Immediately after he left, I climbed the hill to watch him until he disappeared on the horizon. His silhouette carried with it my wildest thoughts and dreams. In the evening after prayers I took a quill and some ink and, by the light of the hearth where a cheerful fire crackled, I tattooed the word *em* on one hand, like an indelible promise. I still bear this mark today but time has made the tattoo pale. In short, I became a *Lhamenpa*.* It happened this way.

In Lhasa, an eminent scholar of Chagpori, Khenrab Norbu, had become the personal physician of the thirteenth Dalai Lama. In the year oxen-water [1913][22] the Prime Minister, Chedra, had gone to the British West Indies. Khenrab Norbu had gone with him to analyze and treat a certain number of illnesses then considered incurable. When foreign doctors, especially British, questioned him on the relationship between the body and the mind with regard to cardiac afflictions, Khenrab Norbu provided extensive detail, as much on the causes as on the symptoms and the psychic consequences related to these pathologies. His visit was a triumph. He was congratulated, photographed and showered with presents. By the time he returned to Tibet his new reputation had preceded him.

Three years later, in the year dragon-fire, 1916, a member of the *Kashag**, the Council of Ministers, asked the thirteenth Dalai Lama, Thoupten Gyatso, for authorization to build a school on the site of the former monastery of Tenguieling, where English would be taught. His request was refused. Then Tekhang Jampa Thoupouang, the personal physician of the Dalai Lama, who became the master of Khenrab Norbu, addressed a request to His Holiness, proposing to build a college of medicine and astrology on the site of the destroyed monastery. The Dalai Lama analyzed all the advantages for rich and poor, aristocrats and peasants, that could result from such an institution, to the point of verifying for himself all the blocks that were used for printing the Gyushi, the texts containing the medical teachings. Then he sent for Tekhang to communicate his agreement. Men-Tsee-Khang, meaning the House of Medicine and Astrology, was thus founded.

When its construction was completed, His Holiness named Tekhang as director of the institute and Khenrab Norbu as principal administrator. In this new establishment the two scholars established the rules and organized the teaching, including the duration of studies, the curriculum, practical applications, examinations, the different levels and classes, the collection of medicinal herbs and the furnishing of other medicinal ingredients, pharmacology and astrology. All of the disciplines were to be taught with equal importance there. It was not surprising that from its beginning the institute acquired considerable notoriety, attracting like a lotus flower carefully selected students from the Tibetan monasteries and the army. Also tantric adepts from Bhutan, Sikkim, Ladakh, Lahaul and Spiti were enrolled, thus illustrating the words of Padma Sambhava*:

> *However removed the place where a savant dwells may be,*
> *His knowledge acts as the messenger.*
> *Like the precious stone of the Ketakai,*
> *He attracts people like bees.*

This is the way it worked. When the Men-Tsee-Khang was ready to recruit students, the Kashang sent a notice to all the monasteries. A single condition for being accepted at the medical institute of Lhasa was that you were under thirteen years of age. Three students at Chothey, among the most brilliant, Yeche Tenzin, Dong-Tchok and Pelden Tseouang, were chosen. But before leaving for Lhasa, the recruits first had to study at the monastery under the direction of a physician, Dr Chekar, who himself had been trained at Men-Tsee-Khang.

Not one of these three students finished his preparation. Yeche Tenzin, the first student with Chekar, ran away from Chothey. Much later I learned that he had hidden among the monks of another monastery, Sera. In turn, Dong-Tchok, a distant relative of my family, disappeared. They said he found refuge in a monastery in Lhasa. He came back to Nyemo after 1959 with a wife and two children. Pelden Tseouang disappeared and was never seen again. Why exactly did they leave? I found out much later through my own experience. Anyway, a doctor wrote a report to Men-Tsee-Khang and chose three other monks. I was among them. Logically, my age should have been a handicap because I was already sixteen but I was considered an intelligent student, sincere and assiduous at work, so an exception was made for me.

The acceptance from Men-Tsee-Khang reached Chothey while I was away reciting prayers for a family. On my return the novices surrounded me to announce that I had been chosen to pursue medical studies. Filled with gladness, I thought I must have accumulated some good karma in my past lives to deserve this; but some of the monks put me on guard, affirming forcefully that becoming an *amchi* carried numerous disadvantages. And then there was Dr Chekar . . .

From the day of my acceptance on, I had to devote myself entirely to my medical studies; no more question of going to families to receit chapten, and games and walks also became rare. Dr Chekar Amchila, was my master in medicine at Chothey and from the beginning I understood why the first students had fled! Besides the sacred texts that had to be learned by heart, I had to do all sorts of jobs that had nothing to do with preparing for my entrance to Men-Tsee-Khang.

Dr Chekar was an unusual man. He took care of his

patients perfectly well; but he gave little attention to his students. Most of my time was spent cleaning his lodging and the attached stables, because he had a passion for horses. When he visited patients outside the monastery, he always went on horseback. As soon as he returned, I had to look after his steed. Later he inspected my work like a military review and incessantly he heaped reproaches on me. Terribly unhappy, I sometimes sought refuge with my tutor. There I endured a second reprimand. As soon as he saw me, he would start scolding me because he did not like the idea of my leaving for Lhasa. His words wounded me:

'You really don't have any good fortune. You lost your mother when you were scarcely born and now you have to work hard for others instead of studying the sacred texts with me. You really have bad karma, Tenzin.'

Maybe he was right. It was already 1939, the year of hare-earth, and I had turned seventeen. Every night I had to get up twice to give fodder to the horses. I would be so exhausted that I was often unable to wake up. *Amchila* knew precisely the time I arrived in the stables because the horses wore little bells and their ringing would wake him.

In the early morning my professor frequently beat me with a whip or a stick before sending me to collect the horse dung and set it out to dry to make manure, which I then had to spread in the nearby fields several times a week.

One day some patients came to consult *Amchila*. They had tied their horses up at the entrance to the monastery, but one of the horses managed to undo the rope that held it and galloped off. At that moment I was in the stable tending to my master's horse. When he was informed of the incident, he accused me of undoing the rope and struck me on the head several times with a stick.

'Tenzin, don't come back here without that horse.'

It was winter, and I started out barefoot in the snow. For a moment I thought luck was with me because the hoof prints were still visible. But as the snow began to fall ever stronger and denser, all traces disappeared in a few hundred meters. That was when I felt the cold overtake me and my feet begin to freeze. With every step I suffered horribly. I was crying, thinking of my *Amala* who was not there to watch over me. Since her death, seventeen years earlier, I had endured much suffering; but this time I did not accept the injustice that I felt I had been dealt. I wandered all day and did not find the horse. The cold and the snow burned my feet to the point that I no longer felt any pain. I had recited the mantra *Om Mani Padme Hum* hundreds of times.

They had assigned a tutor to provide me with an education and a master for my study of medicine, and there I was in the middle of winter, barefoot, looking for a horse that I certainly would never find. I turned around and went back to the monastery. When I found my tutor that night, he flew into a rage:

'I can't get you to study the sacred writings, but others make you work like a dog, like a simple servant.'

That night I could not sleep. I fed the horses and sat down before the altar. The horse's flight, the cold and the snow, my frozen feet and hunger, it all overwhelmed me. Tears rolled freely down my face. I regretted not having left for Lhasa sooner. The more I prayed, the more convinced I became: whether or not I would be happy, I had to enter Men-Tsee-Khang. It had become an imperious necessity.

A few days later there was another incident. Chekar returned very irritated. Immediately he came after me, reproaching me for not having cleaned his lodging well enough.

'Everything is clean, master,' I said to him in a low voice.

He approached the pot of water and pointed to the plank that covered it.

'This is dirty. I can see traces of dust.'

He seized a large copper soup-ladle and struck me violently on the head. I was in pain and an enormous bump appeared. It was the last time he had a chance to strike me. From that day on, I put aside a little of my meager portion of *tsampa* to have the food I would need to get to Lhasa.

That evening I fell asleep with my mind consumed by a single thought: I must leave for Men-Tsee-Khang and become an *amchi*.

5

I Will Be a Doctor

Leaving was all I thought about now. Every day, on the
sly, I put aside small amounts of *tsampa* in a sack that I
hid in a bush. Then I would go into the temple to
perform my rituals. A little off to the side, I meditated
for a long time. The monks there would be saying
prayers uninterrupted, unaware of my intentions. It
was impossible to launch this new adventure without
making minute preparations for the trip. I still had
the burning memory of that Mount Kalaish escapade
that ended with a whipping from my tutor. This time
I would not repeat that mistake. I simply hoped that
Mola would understand and that *Amala* would guide my
steps.

Finally the big day arrived. My tutor had obtained
Chekar's authorization to let me go and recite the
Kanguiour at Cha-Go. I was supposed to come back
in the evening, but the recitations lasted longer than
expected. When I returned to Chothey, it was already
very late; an opportunity like this might not come again
for a long time. Instead of going to my tutor's or my
professor's quarters, I went straight to the hiding place
that held the bundle, the sack of food and a *chupa*.

It must have been about midnight when, armed with my precious booty, I entered the principal temple for the last time.

I pushed open the heavy door that groaned loudly on its hinges. For a few seconds I remained on the threshold to allow the final image I would probably have of the sanctuary of Chothey to penetrate my mind, then I sat down in a dark corner. My eyes met those of the Shakyamuni Buddha, and I was absorbed by it. An intense warmth and emotion filled me as I looked at the butter lamps lined up in their little silver and gold beakers. Before the altar I placed a *kata* and a modest offering of *tsampa*. Some monks were praying and paid no attention to my presence. A good half-hour went by like this. I asked the divinities to crown my enterprise with success and permit me to meet the famous Khenrab Norbu, the personal physician of the Dalai Lama. Appeased, if not serene, I got up and left as discreetly as possible. The temple door closed behind me without making the slightest sound.

Filled with confidence and courage I went toward the principal exit of the monastery, walking on the path that circled the building. I made one more circuit to impregnate myself totally with the holy atmosphere of Chothey, then crossed the gardens and the wooden bridge. With the night and the fury of the water that struck the side of the gorge, I felt an instant's hesitation, but a more powerful force pushed me forward nevertheless. Quickly Chothey disappeared into the dark night behind me.

Soon I arrived at Tachi Noupka, the village where a few of my mother's relatives still lived. Despite the late hour they responded to my knocking. My aunt Pessala had left for Lhasa to attend the festival of *Monlam**, but I found another aunt who was quite fond of me and who regularly worried over my fate.

'There you are in fine clothes. Since your mother died, you've known much suffering, Tenzin. I truly hope you succeed in your endeavor. Tomorrow morning a guide will lead you to Chou. One of your uncles who is a rich farmer lives there. His name is Sena Deundoup Khangsar. Surely he will help you and, especially, give you good advice. You absolutely must find Pessala in Lhasa. Now, go sleep a little because the road will be long.'

My rest was brief but I had a marvelous dream. Many people were entering a monastery while I was blowing into a white conch shell. Later I learned that such a dream is a favorable omen that augurs success. They even say that if you dream it at dawn, great success is certain. Afterwards I slept the sleep of the just.

My aunt awakened me for morning prayers. I abandoned my monastic robe for a *chupa*, swallowed a cup of salted tea and ate a little *tsampa*. The guide was already there. After my aunt had given me a last piece of advice, I fell proudly into step with him. It was five o'clock in the morning.

First we crossed Nyemo, *Amala*'s birth village. Around noon we made a short stop. The guide never exchanged more than a few words with me, only to say that we stilll had to walk four hours to reach Chou. Not much happened in the course of this day, except for our meeting some nuns who belonged to the monastery of Bero. They had filled their buckets in a nearby river and were returning to their convent shrieking with laughter. I concluded that this vision of simple happiness was another favorable omen.

At Chou the guide led me directly to my uncle, Sena Deundoup Khangsar, who offered us tea. I presented him with a *kata*. I found him to be a kind man and very attentive to me.

'When I heard of your mother's death, I thought much about the two children she left, you and your brother. At the time I wasn't able to be of any help to you. Today I'm pleased by your intention to become an *amchi*. But you must learn to be careful. The road to Lhasa is not safe; there is no question of your undertaking this trip alone.'

I spent two nights with my uncle. He checked minutely my newly provisioned bundle that now contained food, warm clothing and shoes. Chou was a large village where the houses were built in tiers on the mountainside. The Khangsar family occupied the highest one. This splendid place looked out onto an immense panorama, a pretty stream, alongside which a twisting road leading to Yang-Chen crossed the valley. A relay stop for merchants, Chou was regularly frequented by caravans. The surrounding hills were covered with green pastures where magnificent horses gamboled in complete freedom. The region greatly resembled Switzerland, which I came to know many years later.

My first day in Chou I told my uncle I felt the need to walk in the hills, and he put me on guard about the dangers of encountering wild animals. A path snaked to the top, cutting across the meadowland. The sun felt like a warm arm across my shoulders and a light breeze played on my face. I was happy, drunk with a freedom I had never known until now. I closed my eyes and held my breath as long as I could. Ah! If *Amala* had only been with me. I would have had so many things to tell her, so much to share! But I was without a mother, and this absence was painful to me. *Om Mani Padme Hum*.

I had almost reached the summit when suddenly I was encircled by a herd of horses led by a stallion whose coat was copper-colored. So as not to frighten them I stood motionless. My heart was almost beating out of my chest. The leader approached in my direction but kept at a distance. He scrutinized me. His hooves struck the earth nervously. He whinnied, and the sound covered the singing of the birds. He snorted, raised his head and whinnied again. Then he came towards me arrogantly, followed by the other horses. As if hypnotized, I could not turn my gaze away. His eyes were burning coals in which the sun's rays sparkled. His ears pointed forward. His mane was raised, floating in the wind, and his tail whipped the air with a wild rhythm. The herd, about ten horses, were close enough to touch me. Somehow I was able to overcome the fear that filled me. The stallion sniffed me and whinnied a last time. All at once he pirouetted and took off at a gallop, followed by the other horses. Their hooves hammered the rocky ground so hard that I felt the vibrations in my body.

After that I decided to rest a little on the heights, and I found a large stone on which to perch and contemplate the valley. In this place the earth touched the sky at an altitude of more than three thousand meters. Crows traced immense circles before alighting in a band on the treetops. Noticing a little grotto, I entered it, assembled a few stones and undertook to build an altar. When, a good hour later, I had finished, I placed an offering there and burned a few juniper twigs. Then I began to recite prayers.

The sun was still high in the sky, so I pushed my exploration further. Here the mountain became more arid. I met nomads with their herds of yaks, *dri* and sheep. Further on behind the grasses, I saw musk deer, chamois and, in the air, eagles. To these I addressed a few words of friendship. As if to let me know he had understood, an enormous male slowly raised his wings and left the ground. He soared high until he was swallowed by the sun and disappeared from my sight. I was thinking of *Mola*, of the hill near my house, and I began to turn in a circle with arms open. I was a bird, and I was free. Milarepa, a saint, hermit and poet, wrote some nine centuries ago:

> *Around me beasts of prey roar,*
> *The royal vulture soars by itself.*
> *The wild ass and the deer play and gambol with their little*
> *   ones,*
> *Larks and white cranes sing all their notes.*

Suddenly a rainbow appeared. I thought again of *Amala*. I began to cry and tears streamed down my face.

My second day at Chou, I walked down to the river's edge. There was no path, and the vegetation was thick. The water was cool and was flowing so slowly that its movement was almost imperceptible. My uncle's dog had followed me, and I spoke to him from time to time, but he scarcely noticed me. We both strolled in a tranquil rhythm. Children were inventing games; lower down, women were working in the fields, talking and laughing. At that moment, I had the feeling that no more suffering could reach me, either in this life or in any other.

I left Chou on the morning of the third day. My uncle had found a caravan that was leaving in the direction of Lhasa and he had asked some of the men of the Ja-Dong family to look after me. We exchanged *katas* and he gave me more advice.

'I feel much gratitude toward your family,' I said to Sena Deundoup Khangsar. 'You have treated me with such compassion and goodness that I will never forget it. When I am in Lhasa, I will pray for your long life.'

We set out early in the morning. The convoy made its way around the mountain that I had partly climbed the day before, crossed a pass and came back down in the direction of a place called Kar-Khang where only some nomads were living. They had set up their tents around an immense fire. This is where we spent the night. The sky had become very dark, but the vastness could still be felt in the mountains. If the days were relatively warm, the evenings were rather cool, and the nights were glacial. I was not dressed to withstand such temperature differences. The eldest of the Ja-Dong family explained to the chief of the nomads that it would be better for me to sleep inside one of the tents and invited me into his family's tent. There they installed me in the most sheltered part because that night a strong wind was sweeping the slope. My escorts from the caravan slept outside in what we call a *kiok-kiok*, a sort of enclosure fabricated by piling up dung and mud. The Ja-Dongs found refuge there for themselves and their animals.

It was to *Mola* that my thoughts flew that night. I even dreamed that we were going somewhere together in a place that seemed to me very dark. *Mola* had raised me in the absence of my mother, had lent me her support when I went to Chothey, and now to Men-Tsee-Khang. I owed her so much. What to say of *Pala*? He preferred the children that his second wife had given him, especially the girls to whom he gave turquoise and coral jewelry. I could not hold that against him, but he might have given my brother and me a little more love and attention. In spite of my suffering, I assured myself of auspicious omens: first, that dream in the course of which I had blown into a shell, then the encounter with the nuns, and, on the road from Chou to Kar-Khang, the donkeys which were carrying innumerable empty pots. Later when I was in prison under the Chinese occupation I had occasion to reflect on all that. I decided then to save as much as possible out of the little that I owned to buy a large silver bowl that would be used for lighting the butter lamps, which are an aid for reflecting on the impermanence of life. When in 1980 I proposed to give it to Jetsune Pema, His Holiness's younger sister, who was on a mission in Tibet, she told me that the transport of such a cumbersome object would not be possible. So I placed it on an altar of the Jokhang*, the principal temple of Lhasa, along with that of Ramotche, and it may still be there today, provided the Chinese have not stolen it.

When I woke up it was still dark but the camp was lively. I heard the crackling of the fire and the hum of the nomads reciting their early morning prayers.

The next day was also long. The caravan advanced slowly. After leaving Kar-Khang, we had to cross a pass and climb the side of a mountain. On the right side, the green waters of a lake shimmered and the valley was calm and peaceful. We progressed with difficulty on a narrow rocky path. The donkeys slipped frequently and we had to hold onto them to keep them from falling into the void. Their hooves made a hollow sound. Rocks broke loose and rolled like thunder to the bottom of the gorge and whole slabs of snow fell away from the mountain walls. Finally managing to traverse this difficult passage, we reached a valley where we did not meet another living being for several hours. When we arrived at Tsourpou, we were welcomed but scarcely installed in the guest quarters when some donkey-drivers arrived. They came from Lhasa, the 'city of the gods'. That evening, I prayed for a long time before the altar and the statue of the Shakyamuni Buddha and offered a *kata* and a little *tsampa*.

The next day was without problems. We stopped around eight o'clock to drink some tea. The sun pierced the sky above the mountains but it was extremely cold. When the caravan started out again, we had to cross a new pass, approaching the eternal snows. Breathing became more and more labored. Finally, we found a valley that led us to Nang-Tse, where we stopped for the night. The following day we would reach Lhasa and my exitement was high. The last day led us to Cha-Ta, in the area of which the family of the caravan lived. After I had rested a little, they escorted me to Lou-Bouk, the part of Lhasa where my aunt Pessala was staying.

The city was lively. It was in the middle of the festival of *Monlam* and I had never seen so many people. Everywhere there were monks and men and women from all the regions of Tibet. The Ja-Dongs explained to me that the first two days were celebrated by the government and the lay people. The *Monlam Chenmo** began on the morning of the third day. For this part, monks and pilgrims filled the capital, whose population quadrupled. It was practically impossible to get near Jokhang or any of the other temples.

My aunt Pessala welcomed me with open arms. We shared tea and made offerings. Now that I was in Lhasa I had to find an opportunity for an introduction at Men-Tsee-Khang and, if possible, a meeting with the great master Khenrab Norbu. Going there during *Monlam* was out of the question.

'The city will be calm again in the next few days,' my aunt told me. 'Then it will be the time for you. The Men-Tsee-Khang is an important institution. Getting admitted there will be difficult, Tenzin, because you have nothing. I advise you to invoke the deities' help from here on.'

Pessala was right. Well, I had to discover Lhasa and this is how I threw myself into the exploration. There was a succession of ceremonies. In this year dragon-fire (1940), which is important in the history of Tibet, the population was euphoric. They had just participated in the installation of Lhamo Theundroup[23]. Some monks told me how the 'chosen child' had arrived in Lhasa, seated on a *trel-lam*, which was a sort of seat attached to two poles and tied to two mules. An immense crowd had come to welcome its new Dalai Lama. Since this day, Lhasa had been celebrating. They intoned songs of welcome, danced and especially prayed. The Tibetans, men, women, and children, were dressed in their best outfits. You heard people crying: 'The day of our happiness has arrived.' The rich aristocrats organized refined evening parties. There were numerous dance and opera performances. I kept thinking how lucky I was because, in Tibet, the majority of the population had never seen the 'city of the gods'. Nomads and farmers worked the earth and pastured their flocks. Monks lived a strict monastic life, sometimes without ever seeing or hearing what went on elsewhere. Needless to say, everything that I had ever heard about Lhasa stirred my curiosity. Besides, arriving in Lhasa a few days after Kundun could only be favorable to me.

The day began at four o'clock, with a short pause at sunrise. The inhabitants of Lhasa brought their contributions to the monks, serving them tea mixed with *tsampa* and a rice-based soup enriched with meat, butter, dried fruits and cheese. An important moment of *Monlam* was the *Soung Cheura*. The monks who had finished their studies attempted to obtain the title of *lharampa*, doctor of philosophy. These philosophical jousts always drew crowds. The superiors of the monasteries were present, and a jury decided the grade to award each participant. But already *Tsok-Cheu Monlam* was coming to an end. This second part, twelve days after the preceding one, was the occasion for new debates of logic, during which the monks tried to obtain the title of *tsokrampa**, doctor of the second degree. In the meantime, the Tibetans continued to demonstrate their joy before the Potala, the Dalai Lama's residence, while the monks exhibited the flags and banners of the different monasteries. In a few days Lhasa emptied out. Tradition required that, before leaving, each monk throw a stone into the river to reinforce the dam. The inhabitants put away their special clothing and the city recovered its usual calm. I was very impressed and in the evening before going to sleep I asked myself if there existed elsewhere in this world other cities larger and more beautiful than Lhasa.

74

I took advantage of the festival to visit the principal temple of the city, Jokhang, and practice devotions. For the first time I saw Joo, the representation of the Shakyamuni Buddha, the most venerated deity of Tibet. Before his altar, strongly imploring my admission to Men-Tsee-Khang, I experienced contrasting emotions, from deep joy to anguish. Every evening I returned from my devotions to Pessala. We spoke a lot about our family and invoked, not without fear, my future. She advised me to visit a certain lama, a distant relative on my maternal side.

'He is a good man who one day left the imprint of his finger on a rock. He knows Men-Tsee-Khang well; perhaps he would provide good advice?'

The next day Pessala brought me to him. Incense was burning on an altar in a corner of the room we entered. We found the lama seated on a little throne, and we presented him with a *kata*. Pessala spoke to him about me for a long time, about my birth, the death of *Amala*, and my wish to become an *amchi*. She also explained to him that I had not had the opportunity to learn much, my professors having used me mostly for menial labor. Finally, she implored his help.

'To become an *amchi*, you will have to make great efforts and develop a solid energy in order to surmount the difficulties. Remember this story, Tenzin. There was once a lama who meditated in an isolated place. At the entrance to the grotto, where he had taken up his retreat, there was a thorn bush which hooked his clothes every time he entered or left. "I must cut that bush," he would say to himself, but he did nothing about it. Because he was reflecting on impermanence and death, this idea left him and he returned to his practice. When he had finished his retreat, the bush was still in the same place, but the man had become a wise and accomplished master. You see, Tenzin, even if I know the director of Men-Tsee-Khang, you have absolutely no need of my help.'

Hearing these words, I became angry. I think I must have been positively insolent because I had placed so much hope in this meeting. I left without even turning around, while Pessala continued to implore the lama. Later, on the way back home, she reprimanded me justifiably: my behavior had been utterly unworthy of a monk.

'You have no manners, Tenzin.'

'I don't need the lama to become an *amchi*.' I shot back at her. 'I don't want to wait any longer. Tomorrow, I will go to Men-Tsee-Khang by myself and nothing will be able to change my decision.'

That evening I spent a long time before the altar, hoping that a dream of good omen would come to me as I slept. And this is the dream that came: I was in a room where two professors of medicine were seated; one was old, the other younger. The latter was speaking to me, affirming that I was an ideal person for this work. When I awoke, I believed that this dream was really not a good omen and that my immediate future would continue with menial labor. The dream actually meant no such thing as I was soon going to discover.

One last time Pessala put me on guard: I would pay for my insolence and, especially, I would find no-one to grant my request. I pretended not to hear her. As I had nothing else to offer, I brought a *kata*.

Men-Tsee-Khang was not far from Lou-Bouk and a

road led directly there. I walked quickly and my mind was in turmoil, halfway between doubt and hope.

For the first time I entered Men-Tsee-Khang. It was nine o'clock, and patients were already there. I let the attendants think I was ill. I waited almost two hours before my turn came. Two men were standing in the room. One was much older than the other. He gestured to me to sit down. At the instant he was going to take my pulse, I said to him:

'I am not ill, *amchila*. My name is Tenzin Choedrak. I have come from the monastery of Chothey and I want to become an *amchi* like you. If I hadn't signed in as a patient, they would not have let me meet you.'

'Why have you left Chothey?' he asked me.

'My professor would often leave to care for patients. His prolonged absences did not allow me to learn suitably.'

Fearing abrupt dismissal, I voluntarily omitted speaking to him of the many duties to which Dr Chekar had assigned me. The two men were staring at me now with perplexed expressions.

'Permit me to study at Men-Tsee-Khang with the master, Khenrab Norbu. *Lhamenpa* has always been an example for me, and that is the only reason I fled here from Chothey.'

'But you know that leaving like that is an affront to your professor. You have acted badly, Tenzin Choedrak, and by your behavior you have insulted him,' the older man said to me in a severe tone.

It was now that I realized that the two men standing next to each other here were exactly as those in my dream. The one speaking to me resembled a bodhisattva. His speech was direct, and his words rang true, even if they wounded me terribly.

'Before you, three other novices have already fled from Chothey,' remarked the younger man.

Until then, he had not said a word to me, but he had never taken his eyes off me, scrutinizing my every gesture, analyzing each of my words, each sentence.

'We cannot make a decision today,' he finally said to me. 'Come back tomorrow, Tenzin Choedrak, and we will advise you.'

The younger man, the one who had just spoken to me, was none other than the personal physician[24] of Kundun, who was then five years old and had just arrived in Lhasa. He also bore the title of *Lhamenpa*.

When I returned to Lou-Bouk, I related my adventure to Pessala and shared with her my wild hopes.

'Be confident, Tenzin. Remember the lama's story.'

The next day, I rushed to Men-Tsee-Khang. The two men were there. This time it was the *Lhamenpa* who spoke to me.

'We have decided, Tenzin Choedrak, to accept you into our institute. As custom requires, you must offer the tea ceremony. Do you have any family in Lhasa?'

An intense joy overwhelmed me. I explained that my aunt Pessala was living for the moment in the city.

'But you told us yesterday that you possessed nothing. How will you manage, Tenzin?'

'I will borrow the money from Pessala.'

'Does she have any money to spare?'

'I don't know, *Lhamenpa*. If she doesn't, perhaps she could borrow some? Please, don't refuse me.'

Briefly the two men consulted each other with a look.

'So be it,' said *Lhamenpa*. 'Here is the list of the estimated expenses for your admission to Men-Tsee-Khang.'

For the time the sum was of consequence. I had to find five *dotse*[25], the equivalent today of three thousand Indian rupees. Pessala borrowed the money from one of her acquaintances at ten per cent interest. I pledged to reimburse her for everything. To do this, I sent a letter to my uncle the tutor, announcing my admission and explaining that I was going to take care of the tea offering myself. A few months later I received a message from him and the amount which he had somehow been able to put together. I was most grateful to him because I knew he had only enough for his own basic needs. His gift enabled me to pay Pessala back.

Finally, the tea ceremony known as *Tong-Go* took place. I was anxious, but it all went well. I had bought two bricks of tea in sheets, ten kilos of *dri* buter, and a large quantity of rice, for all of which five *dotse* was enough. I offered the tea and some *dre-sil*, a plate of sugared rice, to a good sixty students and envelopes containing a little money to four or five professors.

Since I was poor, I had bought a cheaper grade of tea. There was another one of better quality, which at the time cost the equivalent of fifty rupees. Usually this tea took on a bright red color when infused. A strange thing now happened. When I served my tea, it had taken on the appearance of the better tea. All the students commented on the event. For me it was another good omen which, as we now know, signified that I would become an *amchi*.

I was now a student at Men-Tsee-Khang, and I promised myself to study very hard. That night sleep came to me late. As I lay awake, I made an offering to Tara and addressed this tribute to her:

Homage to you, Tara, Liberator, quick and intrepid,
Your expression is bright like lightning,
You appeared in an opened flower,
From a tear on the face of the Lord of the three worlds

Praise to you, whose face shines
With a brightness like that of a hundred full moons of
  autumn,
You cast a clear and splendid light
More intense than that of a thousand stars.

6

'I Bow Before You and All the Buddhas'

It was now the early 1940s. I devoted my days to studying. At the time I had hardly any interest in politics. It was said that Tibetan society was seeking to open itself to the outside world. Lhasa was rife with rumors, and there were strong tensions between the aristocrats and the religious. I, however, was a hundred leagues from being able to imagine the events that were taking place in the capital, in Tibet as a whole, and certainly even less outside the country[26]. I had come here to learn medicine, and nothing else mattered to me.

After my admission I left Pessala's home for a room at Men-Tsee-Khang that I shared with four other students. Lodging conditions were miserable. They allotted us thin mattresses, and since the floor was always damp, in the morning we had to dry them out to be able to sleep on them again in the evening. Because I had no money, I had to sell two or three porcelain bowls that I owned, keeping only a single one that was chipped. This gave me a small sum that allowed me to buy the books required for my studies. Neither the obstacles I encountered nor the lack of comfort turned me from my objective. And I felt an even greater pride in having been admitted to the institution directed by the Venerable Khenrab Norbu.

The days were very regimented for the sixty to seventy students. At four o'clock in the morning a trumpet awakened us and we had only a few minutes to get to the hall for prayers. We would first invoke Manjoushri, the manifestation of the wisdom of all the Buddhas[27], and then Tara:

> *Hail to you whose body is blue and gold,*
> *Your hands perfectly ornamented with the lotus,*
> *You who are generosity, energy, asceticism, peace,*
> *Patience, concentration and wisdom.*

> *Hail to you, who like the ouchincha, crown of all the*
> * Buddhas,*
> *Enjoy complete victory over numberless obstacles.*
> *The bodhisattvas, who have sublimated perfection*
> *Show you great veneration.*

Then there followed a ceremony during which we burned incense. After this, each of us spent an hour studying with his professor, who explained the section of the texts learned that morning so we would have the clearest possible understanding. The operational tasks were performed by turns. Lunch was prepared by the students themselves, who were for the time let out of class for this purpose. The meals were mostly radishes and potatoes cut into pieces and cooked with a meager amount of meat and mixed with tea, butter and some *tsampa*.

After lunch we had two hours of calligraphy. We had to recopy fragments of the texts we had studied with the professors. We would have to write twelve lines a day, which naturally had to be acceptable to the professor, who was extremely severe. There was a break around four o'clock. Immediately after this short rest, we had to memorize the texts on which we would be questioned the next morning. Then we had to memorize medical texts until six o'clock. This was a nerve-wracking exercise for all of us. When this work session ended, we would pass in turn before the professor to recite what we had learned. A modest student, it was at the price of considerable effort that I succeeded in retaining three, sometimes four pages, while the most brilliant among us would be able to retain five or six pages. It was not unusual for some of us to be punished by being deprived of the morning meal. The others would make fun of us, with remarks like: 'I see you're not eating!' 'So you're not hungry today?' The memorizing usually ended around six o'clock, but sometimes later. Only then could we think about dinner, which lasted barely a half-hour. The day was still not over. We would go up to the terrace until nine o'clock, and sometimes even eleven o'clock. Seated in groups of three or four according to the level of our knowledge, we would apply ourselves to reciting texts, which sounded like the recitation of prayers. In fact, this reading sharpened our memory. We had one day off a week, Sunday. The morning of that day, we had to respond successfully to an oral questioning on everything we had studied in the course of the previous days. Those who answered incorrectly were not allowed to leave Men-Tsee-Khang and the professors did not hesitate to crack the whip on them. Those who recited to the satisfaction of our professors were free to go out a little or to wash their clothes. In the evening of our day off another debating session awaited us.

The moment has come for me to describe the person who was my master at Men-Tsee-Khang, Khenrab Norbu. I have recounted as faithfully as possible the words pronounced by him during the inestimable moments that I spent in his company. I might have called this phase of my story 'Cloud of offerings to the eternally prosperous Master of medicine'. I address this prayer to him as a simple homage to his memory.

> *On the celestial path of the compassion and knowledge of all*
>   *the Buddhas,*
> *Benefactor who cured ignorance and illness,*
> *May the Medicine Buddha triumph over all.*
> *In the countries of the Teaching of the Buddha,*
> *Which has flourished here as nowhere else,*
> *From the Wheel of Existence you appeared as a being*
>   *capable of enlightening*
> *People about their good and bad actions.*
> *You studied astrology and medicine in depth for many*
>   *years,*
> *Then accomplished a work vast as the sky.*
> *You have spread the practice*
> *And helped the ignorant and those who fear death.*
> *You were a fine professor of medicine and astrology.*
> *To you, excellent Khenrab Norbu, I render homage.*
> *I bow before you and all the other Buddhas.*

I did not compose this prayer in order to satisfy my pride, but to answer the requests of my own students. My master's teachings remain engraved in the depths of my mind. His life was exemplary.

A famous astrologer, Trang Goleb, and his wife, Yangtchen, lived in the city of Tsethang in the heart of the Valley of the Kings. They had two children, the eldest of whom, Khenrab Ouangthcouk, entered the monastery of Drepoung when he was still a child. Khenrab Norbu was the younger child.

On the day of his birth the full moon directed all its light on the child's head, which could have signified that one day the little Khenrab Norbu would possess the ability to effect good all around him. His father showed him special attention, taking him everywhere with him. The young Khenrab adored these shared moments, especially when his father went into homes to perform astrological readings. Their influence not only in the practice of medicine but in the daily lives of Tibetans cannot be emphasized enough.

According to his family's wishes, the child entered the monastery of Ngachod at Tsethang. He was soon noticed for his intelligence and his goodness. When he would go to fetch water from the river, Khenrab Norbu loved to look enviously at the fruits ripening in the trees in the summer sun, especially the apricots, the sight of which made him happy. Many years later after he had become the physician of the thirteenth Dalai Lama, Khenrab Norbu had numerous apricot trees planted in the garden of his residences at Men-Tsee-Khang and Bha-ra-Lhu-go. 'A childhood memory,' he would say, laughing.

Scarcely thirteen years old, Khenrab Norbu entered the monastery of Chagpori. His mother, who tended to him closely, offered to accompany him as far as Lhasa. But the child was not to travel alone; another novice was also to go to the monastery of Ganden[28] to continue his education. They made the trip together seated on the back of a mare. A sincere friendship was born between the two boys, and when they parted, they promised each other that they would study hard.

'One day, I'll be a *Lhamenpa*,' Khenrab joked, laughing.

'And me, I'll become a *Ganden Tripa*[29],' said the novice.

The years went by, and their jokes came to pass.

Chagpori did not seem strange to Khenrab Norbu. Perhaps he had a memory of it from one of his earlier lives. The interiors of the buildings were familiar to him and he thought he recognized the immediate area. He began to study under the direction of Ngaouang Sera, the doctor of the monastery of Sera. In order to perfect himself in his apprenticeship, and applying to the letter the directions contained in the text of the *Four Tantras*, the *Gyushi**, he even went to collect the excrement of his old professor, Kelsang, to practice analysis.

Up early and to bed late, Khenrab memorized the texts much faster than the other students. Morning and evening he would go to fetch the water from the river and light the fire. When there were festivities in Lhasa, he did not linger in the city. He showed little interest in his clothes, hardly taking the time to mend his monastic robe. With the help of a string, he was content to make innumerable knots to keep together what soon became rags. Because of that, he was nicknamed 'Hundred Knots of Ngachod'.

Khenrab Norbu rapidly mastered the basic texts of Tibetan medicine and passed all his examinations without difficulty. He looked for a professor qualified to help him advance still further in his studies, and he longed to work under the direction of the personal physician of His Holiness the thirteenth Dalai Lama.

It was thus that, several times, Khenrab Norbu solicited one of the most renowned physicians, Tekhang Jampa Thoupouang. On each of his visits to him, he spoke to him of his passion for medicine and his wish to meet the best professors. Tekhang did not immediately show outwardly the interest that he had in this adolescent monk who did not hesitate to pester him at every moment. One day, however, when he received the young Khenrab, he offered him a *kata* and some butter and asked him to come back the next day, promising to give him all the teachings that he was demanding with such insistence.

The student showed himself more and more assiduous and questioned Tekhang not only about the *Four Tantras* but also culture and civilization. Thus by this rare flowing of benedictions and signs of good omen, Tekhang Jampa Thoupouang poured little by little an ocean of knowledge into Khenrab Norbu.

It was a tradition that Chagpori required the students to go and work as assistants for six months at the temple of Jokhang. When young Khenrab's turn came, he refused to renounce his meetings with the master early in the morning. One day he made the acquaintance of a lama who was living in the grotto of Tamdine and who came regularly to Jokhang. They spoke about medicine and the man said to him:

'I see, Khenrab Norbu, that you work with much energy. However, reading the tantras is not enough to become a master in medicine. It is necessary also to learn grammar and poetry, and in a manner to understand the nuances better.'

Khenrab observed the lama intently.

'Would you agree to be my professor?' he asked him.

The lama agreed to the request and met with him a few days later. When Khenrab Norbu arrived at the grotto of Tamdine, the monk was waiting for him, seated cross-legged on a cushion. Two bowls had been placed on a low table. When the student presented himself, the lama said to him:

'Sit down opposite me, there on that cushion. As it is never good to dispense a teaching to someone who has an empty stomach, we will each drink a bowl of curdled milk.'

In acting thus, the lama was respecting on the one hand, tradition and, on the other, reuniting good auspices. The lama then began his teaching on the bases of the *Soumtchoupa* and the *Takdjoukpa*, the treatises of grammar. Khenrab Norbu having later become in his turn a great master of Tibetan medicine, he counseled his students never to neglect any discipline, and he would willingly tell them of this incident:

'When the lama was dispensing his teachings to me, he asked me if I knew how to write. "Not very well, master," I answered him. "But I think I'm able to copy any text."

"How can you claim such a thing, Khenrab Norbu? You have just irritated the goddess Yangthcen Lhamo, and you're probably going to bring thunderbolts down on you." '

His entire life Khenrab Norbu remembered the lama's remark, for, despite all his efforts, his calligraphy never improved.

When Tekhang learned about his student's meetings with the lama, he was delighted and advised him to push his learning even further by studying astrology, and Khenrab Norbu duly embarked on it under the guidance of three great masters. When he did not succeed in grasping the deeper meaning and the nuances of a teaching, he would punish himself by buying himself some bread and remaining seated for hours in reflection near a pillar of the temple. On the other hand, when he passed an examination with success, he would readily buy himself a succulent meal in an inn. Sometimes it happened that he forgot to drink the tea served him by the innkeeper. Then it would be served specially to him in his room. In a word, Khenrab Norbu was so determined that he soon had medicine, astrology, grammar, and poetry at his fingertips[30].

In 1908, the year monkey-earth, Khenrab Norbu had turned twenty-five when, during the festival of *Monlam*, a serious epidemic struck the population of Lhasa. He immediately brought his aid and knowledge to the battle against the spread of the virus. Alerted to the exceptional qualities of this young physician, the thirteenth Dalai Lama was also pleased by the tenacity of Khenrab Norbu in wanting to help others. Four years later, in the year mouse-water (1912). he was appointed the resident physician at the monastery of Drepoung. Here he was able to develop different skills, among them the editing of works on astrology and medicine. He showed his works to one of his professors, Dordje Guieltsen, who made some suggestions to refine them even further.

One day when he was completing the calligraphy of some texts essential for his research, Khenrab placed the heavy manuscript on a window sill. A sudden gust of wind scattered his precious work. Without being in the least disturbed, he called to the rescue all the monks in the area. The catastrophe barely averted, it still took him more than a week to reassemble the pages. Later, when he had finished his studies on thirty-seven species of the rarest medicinal plants[31] that could generally be gathered only in the least accessible parts of our mountains, suddenly some began to grow near his residence. Such favorable signs led Khenrab Norbu, always desirous of making his contribution to the evolution and improvement of the health of others, to open a school, the Men-Tsee-Khang, where up to three hundred students would be able to follow his teachings.

During his stay at Drepoung, the Dalai Lama asked him to go to Sikkim to care for the king, who was suffering at the time from an unknown illness. Before his departure, Khenrab Norbu made numerous astrological calculations to determine whether he should meet the ailing sovereign. What he concluded from his readings was of extreme gravity: he would never see the face of the sovereign. He hurried to inform His Holiness Thoupten Gyatso, who refused to take into account the warnings of his doctor and enjoined him to hurry. But when Khenrab Norbu arrived at Nakartse, he learned of the death of the king. He had not been mistaken.

In 1918, the year horse-earth of the Tibetan calendar, Khenrab Norbu became *Lhamenpa*, the personal physician of the thirteenth Dalai Lama. He succeeded Jaboug Damtcheu Peldjor, then too old to continue to occupy such a delicate function.

Every day he rose at three o'clock in the morning, arranged his room, prepared his altar and repeated his lengthy prayers.[32] It was only after that he began his teachings. Then he would proceed, accompanied by two students, to the consulting room where he would calmly treat all the patients. For those who suffered from eye problems he intervened himself in this sensitive zone or asked some students to take over, but only provided they had already been prepared a long time by practicing on a sheep head. After lunch he read texts in his quarters, then visited high government functionaries and aristocrats to prepare their astrological readings.

In the evening after dinner he took walks. He had also developed the habit of caring for sick beggars near the temple of Ramotche*; he would give them *tsampa*, sometimes a little money. He even gave some of his income to the neediest monasteries. Before going to sleep, Khenrab Norbu still found the strength to pray to the protecting deities of medicine and astrology and to teach students about the positions of the stars and the movement of the planets.

At the time the *Kashag* took a more lenient attitude toward the slaughter of animals, and many nomads came to the capital to sell their livestock. The Venerable Khenrab Norbu disliked the idea of killing animals even for food, so he regularly bought yaks and sheep that he saved from death and allowed them to graze in freedom within the wall of Men-Tsee-Khang. There is a Tibetan proverb:

A being of such value and knowledge
Does not lose his learning despite occasional reversals.
The sun, with its burning rays,
Cannot change the cold of the snow.

And then arrived the eighth month of the year monkey-water (1932). On the instruction of the Dalai Lama, Khenrab Norbu was transferred to the monastery of Ngachod at Tsekhang where, on his arrival, he was relieved of his functions of *Lhamenpa*. He was told, however, that he was to keep the administration of Men-Tsee-Khang. In the beginning he did not understand the meaning of this sudden change. Certainly he was aware that an incurable illness, the result of profound sadness and unremitting fatigue, was afflicting His Holiness Thoupten Gyatso and that the cause was his concern for the future of the Tibetans.

At that time the Dalai Lama wrote in his political testament: 'It is certain we are entering a period of oppression and terror, when the days and the nights will be made endless with suffering.'

The sovereign was afflicted by a slight chill, but he nevertheless agreed to participate in certain end-of-the-year ceremonies. In the course of one of them his condition worsened, and he was unable to preside over the *Ganden Ngamtcheu*, the anniversary of the death of Je Tsongkhapa, the founder of the *geloukpa* school. This occurred on the twenty-fifth day of the tenth month of the year bird-water (12 December, 1933). Just the day before, the Dalai Lama had received in audience the monks of the tantric college of Guiume. But that morning, while the day was scarcely dawning over Lhasa, the monks were informed that the sovereign would be unable to participate in the public audience to which they had been invited. In its place there was an audience in the throne room, what we Tibetans call the 'invitation of the robe', during which prayers and chants were recited before the ceremonial robe of the Dalai Lama, which was spread out on his throne.

Five days later, on the evening of the thirtieth day of the year bird-water (17 December, 1933), Thoupten Gyatso left his earthly form. He was fifty-nine years old and had realized to the letter the prediction set forth a year earlier in his political testament. The Tibetans began a long period of mourning, forty-nine days during which the days and nights were devoted to meditation. The Dalai Lama's Palace in Lhasa, the Potala, burned with a thousand flames. According to custom at the time of funeral ceremonies or celebrations of the anniversary of a death, butter lamps were placed outside and on the roofs.

A rumor was growing and there was talk of black magic and poisonings. It was only then that Khenrab Norbu understood why the Dalai Lama had relieved him of his duties as *Lhamenpa*. Having decided to rejoin the 'celestial domains', the Dalai Lama wanted to protect his physician from all suspicion by distancing him from the palace intrigues that would certainly follow his death, by sending him away to the monastery of Ngachod at Tsekhang.

When he was sixty years old, in the year dragon-iron (1940), Khenrab Norbu wanted to know how much time remained to him. To this end he made many astrological calculations. Finally certain that he was not in error, he knew he would leave this life that same year. From that moment on he devoted all his time to his students, of whom I was one, anticipating our future. He made donations to the most impoverished monasteries. Finally, he refused to participate in any more ceremonies, even the most important ones. To keep harm at bay with the hope of extending his life, Khenrab Norbu had a new grotto for the guardian divinity Tagdongchen built at Bar Lougoug. Sculptors were brought in to create a statue of the deity Tamdine Yansang. The deity had always been depicted with a feminine face, but one morning, in Khenrab Norbu's presence, they removed the tiger skin from the unfinished sculpture and they saw an enormous penis. From then on the deity was represented with a masculine face.

Khenrab also had built a miniature Chambhala, in which he was depicted as surrounded by his students and numerous celestial creatures.

'That will bring you luck,' he said to us. 'Myself, I will be reborn at Chambhala, or in the heart of an enchanted medical community.'

Scarcely a year had gone by. One morning at daybreak, leaving a retreat that had lasted several weeks, Khenrab Norbu again invoked the protecting divinities of medicine and astrology with several prayers. Then he drank a cup of tea and decided to leave his residence of Bar Lougoug to return to Men-Tsee-Khang. On the way he made a brief courtesy visit to the oracle of *Netchoung**, and just after this encounter two strange things happened. Khenrab Norbu had a vision of a magnificent city of medicine that shone with a thousand flames in the center of a double rainbow. Just then a piece of paper fell from the sky and turned three times above his head before landing at his feet. He picked it up and unfolded it and there he read the following message: 'You will live to the age of eighty-one.' The master could not believe his eyes, so in contradiction was this to his astrological calculations. When he returned to Men-Tsee-Khang, he wanted to reread the astonishing message that had been addressed to him, but the piece of paper had disappeared. Suddenly he remembered that the Buddha himself had lived to this advanced age. Since this was how it was to be, he realized he had better continue the work he had begun. This was unhoped for. He would be able to see his students put his teachings into practice. A delighted smile spread across his lips. This demonstrates how extraordinary the Venerable One was. He had come into this world to assuage suffering and ignorance and was going to do so for a long time.

More than ten years went by. It was the year dragon-water (1952) or serpent-fire (1953). Tenzin Gyatso, the fourteenth Dalai Lama, reigned over the country. In the year hare-fire (1951), exceptional circumstances had obliged the government to confer temporal powers on him because Communist China had invaded the eastern provinces of Tibet, and for two years the Land of Snows had suffered the worst atrocities.

At this time the *Kashag* received a letter from Chigatse, informing them that an exceptional child had been born to a couple, Gokyd and Azom. The baby bore on its head the pattern of a crown of lotus, and he was found holding in his hand a *vajra*, a white conch shell. The *Kashag* asked Khenrab Norbu to plot the child's astrological chart. In spite of all the care that he brought to his calculations, Khenrab found nothing unusual. A few months later it was discovered that the parents had orchestrated a scene around their child so that it would be thought that he was a reincarnation.* From his birth they had placed little *vajras* in the baby's hands and put one of these shells on a cushion near him. Thanks to Khenrab Norbu, no-one was deceived by this shameful stratagem.

In 1954 (the year horse-wood) just before the Dalai Lama, who was then nineteen years old, was preparing to depart for China, Khenrab Norbu was called to take the pulse of Thoupten Lhundoup, the doctor who was supposed to accompany His Holiness. A short time after this, he confided to friends that the doctor would not survive this trip. The prediction proved to be so accurate that on the Tibetan sovereign's return to the Potala, Khenrab Norbu was called to the bedside of the doctor, who died a few days later, exhausted by the long trip into China and back. Khenrab Norbu had great feeling for Tenzin Gyatso. The young Kundun gave off such an air of serenity that one could not but be touched by it. In spite of his very young age, the Dalai Lama displayed much skill in the face of the Communist occupiers and the events then taking place in Tibet. Khenrab Norbu took great care over Kundun's health. He had begun to trace the evolution of His Holiness from the time he was six years old. Every day, the master redrafted His Holiness's astrological chart, modifying it with other information, some medical, and redid his calculations several times to verify them. All the details of the life of Tenzin Gyatso were accumulating in the many pages written in the astrologer-physician's still unreadable handwriting. Nothing escaped him. Thus it was that Khenrab Norbu knew before the rest of the world that the fourteenth Dalai Lama would become a great spiritual master who would guide the world on a better path. Rather than broadcast such information, which could have incited crazed attacks from the Chinese, the Venerable One again displayed incomparable wisdom by keeping quiet.

Khenrab Norbu rejoined the 'celestial domains' on the twenty-eighth day of the year tiger-water (October, 1962). Today I dedicate this prayer to him:

> *All the acts accomplished by a being such as you*
> *Cannot be understood by beings such as us.*
> *Who would not wish to follow your path,*
> *Engage in an activity such as yours?*
> *May the virtues and the merits assembled*
> *Be dedicated to you.*

7

Student of Tibetan Medicine

I followed my studies with the Venerable Khenrab Norbu. I did not have his abilities and could not immediately assimilate everything that he said to me, but each of his teachings held a great richness for me. Tibetan medicine is part of one of the most ancient traditions in the world: its healing system is unique because its approach is holistic. Unfortunately ignored by Western specialists out of negligence, out of prejudice, and especially indifference, its survival depends essentially on the work carried out presently in Dharamsala.

The *Gyushi*[33] touches on all aspects of illness and contains all the information necessary to diagnose and treat an illness.[34] It regroups all the original information that came from India, which our scholars augmented with techniques and knowledge that they acquired in neighboring countries.

This is not a medical treatise. However, I wish to present some information succinctly in the following pages. As one of the personal physicians of the Dalai Lama, I necessarily take his pulse every day to follow the evolution of his state of health. This is a diagnostic activity, essential in our medical tradition and of great precision. With my right hand I examine his left pulse, then with my left hand I examine his right pulse. By means of several examinations I make a dozen different analyses. With the upper edge of my right index finger I read everything that concerns his heart; with the inferior edge I analyze his small intestine. With the upper edge of my middle finger, his spleen; with the inferior edge, his stomach; with the superior edge of my ring finger, his left kidney; with the inferior edge, his seminal vesicle.[35] The pulse in his left hand indicates other things to me. With the upper edge of my index finger I read his lungs; with the inferior edge his colon; with the upper edge of my middle finger, his liver; with the inferior edge, his biliary vesicle; with the upper edge of my ring ringer, his right kidney; with the inferior edge, his bladder.

For us Tibetans the analysis of the urine is another means of refining the diagnosis. The sample must be the initial emission of the morning. First we stir and beat it, then let it sit, sometimes tasting it to test its sugar level, notably to look for evidence of diabetes. The examination consists of observing its frothiness, sediments, color, steam and odor. Next it is a question of analyzing all its elements in function of the humors, troubles due to heat or cold and the vital organs. According to the *Gyushi*, when the patient is in perfect health his or her urine is then

> *'of a white color lightly tinted with yellow, like the color of butter freshly melted; it is light; its steam is normal and lasts for a moderate duration after the emission; the bubbles are of moderate quantity; after the dissipation of the odor,*

the sediment is blue, lightly tinted with yellow, neither fine nor thick; the froth is fine and stabilizes once the urine's vapor has disappeared.'

In Tibetan medicine ignorance is perceived as the primordial cause of all physical illnesses and all mental perturbation. This holistic perspective will be applied to the patient's diagnosis and treatment. If a humor is out of balance, illness can occur. The Tibetan physician questions the patient and takes into account his or her daily living patterns, habits, nutrition, and environment to understand the pathology better. The analysis of the body is conducted with the understanding that the physical phenomena exist on the basis of the five elements: earth, fire, air, water and space. An individual is composed of five aggregates: form, sensations, identification, mental and conscious formations. The individual's body is regulated by three humors [*nyepa soum*]: wind [*loung*] represents the vital current; bile [*tripa*] is heat; and phlegm [*peken*] represents the aqueous constituents. With these three humors are associated three disturbing passions: ignorance, anger and desire/attachment.

Astrology is another important factor. In fact, it plays an active and important role in our entire society. It may be consulted on the occasion of a birth, a marriage, when a medical treatment is not successful, and when facing death. Able to provide all sorts of information, it is omnipresent. Tibetan astrology includes three specialties. *Kartsi*, or the white calculations comparable to Western astrology, is the study of the planets and the stars and is derived from two Indian sources, the *Tantra kalachakre* and the *Tantra sarodhaya*. It proposes to study human relationships, son–mother, friend–enemy. *Nagtsi* presents many points in common with the classical Chinese system, relating the five elements to one another and necessitating numerous operations. And finally *yang char*, which is the tantric and secret part of the *kartsi*.

If a medical treatment has been followed for a long time and the cure does not come, the patient may look for another therapy with an astrologer. The Tibetan medical texts mention that the physician may consider the possibility that some illnesses may be caused by spirits or a bad karma. Whether the practitioner is a lay astrologer or a lama, such illnesses cannot be treated except with the support of a specific antidote. Spirits are classed in eight categories, to which are attributed specific prayers. At this level the *yang char* intervenes. The astrologer will determine the therapy most appropriate to the causes of the ills from which the patient suffers. The *Root Tantra* represents with extreme precision the human constitution, healthy or ill, in the form of an Indian fig tree. This *Tree of Health and Illness* has three roots, nine trunks, forty-seven branches, two hundred and twenty-four leaves, two flowers and three fruits. The two flowers represent health and long life. The three fruits indicate spiritual development, riches and happiness.

There are also numerous texts that deal with pharmacology. This is discussed in detail notably in the second *Tantra* of the *Gyushi*. It is also to be found in the medicine mandala*, whose four medicinal mountains indicate the treatment of illnesses of a warm nature, illnesses of a cold nature, all illnesses, and the maintenance in good condition of the six vital functions and the organs. The *Gyushi*, which I studied at Men-Tsee-Khang, emphasizes that medications may be extracted from all the substances of the earth. Needless to say, Khenrab Norbu and all the other professors of medicine taught us the curative virtues of the substances which contain medicinal properties, demanding that we treat them with respect and devotion, like an offering to the deities of medicine and astrology. On this subject the *Gyushi* says:

Earth: heavy, strong, firm, bitter. Its properties combat illnesses related to air.

Water: fresh, transparent, sweet. These properties lubricate, humidify, and calm the system and combat illnesses of the bile.

Fire: lively, hot, light, rough. Its properties produce heat in the body, reinforce the seven constitutive elements, embellish the complexion and combat illnesses related to phlegm.

Air: light, unstable, cold, rough. The properties fortify the body, facilitate physical movement and the distribution of the nutritive elements, and combat illnesses of phlegm combined with a bile disorder.

Space: hollow. It combats illnesses of bile, phlegm and air. All plants and other substances possess the nature of space.

From the year dragon-fire to the year monkey-wood (1940 to 1944), at Men-Tsee-Khang I continued to apply myself wholeheartedly to my studies. Age had brought me more maturity and since most of the students were younger than me, the professors were extremely severe with me. On Sundays we would go out in little groups. We enjoyed strolling in the narrow streets of the Lhasa market between the shops. Personally I loved these moments when I could observe the pilgrims who end-lessly turned their prayer wheels with one hand and with the other said their prayer beads, *Om Mani Padme Hum.* I felt so happy among these ordinary people. An old woman resembling *Mola* never failed to come up to me. I was always overcome with emotion. Smiling, she would hand me a bowl of tea and sometimes we had friendly exchanges.

One day a scuffle broke out between our group and some local youths. The fight became nasty and caused a fire to start in a shop. There was a sudden explosion, apparently firecrackers that wounded some who were nearby. On our return to Men-Tsee-Khang, punishment was immediate in the forms of whips that lashed our bodies. From that Sunday on we were forbidden to stroll in the Lhasa market. I felt miserable, and also a little responsible for not being able to separate the trouble-makers. Such a failure could have cost me dearly, and I dared not imagine my eviction from Men-Tsee-Khang. That evening, after the debates of logic, I isolated myself from the others and climbed up to the terrace where it was cool. A light wind needled my skin. I thought about *Amala* and lost myself in the stars. I began to murmur:

> *Homage to Toure, the terrifying one,*
> *Who triumphs over the most tenacious demons.*
> *Her lotus face marked by anger*
> *Destroys all enemies.*

I now knew the texts of the *Gyushi* sufficiently well to be able to tackle the different aspects of Tibetan medicine with some assurance. As I was rather robust, I was regularly asked to assist, at different times of the year, in the grinding of the medicinal plants. Reserved for the oldest of us, the task proved harsh, and it was often necessary to work at a mortar in pairs. Afterwards I would fall asleep exhausted and dream that I was going up into the mountains to collect plants and roots and flowers.

And then my turn came to actually do this. The collection of medicinal plants took place four times a year, each season offering its particularities and its specific products: the first harvest in February and March at the end of winter; the second in May and June when the flowers and the leaves open wide; the third in August and September for the fruits; and finally the last, in September and October, for the gathering up of the roots, whose properties would then be at their maximum.

All of this deserves much explanation. Let me simply say that a plant continues to evolve. It shares the properties and nature of the five elements that produce it: water brings it the humidity necessary to its evolution; warmth supports its development; the air breathes growth into it; and space offers its field for blooming. At the moment the sap rises in a growing plant all the energy becomes concentrated in the upper parts, where the substances that interest us are contained. When the plant reaches maturity, its energy is displaced to become concentrated in its seeds and leaves. Then a few months later its fruits will furnish the ingredients necessary to certain medications. Finally, when the plant dies, we utilize its roots. A single species may possess different properties according to the stage of its development, and distinct flavours depending on when it is harvested.

It is sugary when earth and water predominate, like saffron, butter, honey, meat; acid when earth and fire predominate, like yogurt or yeast; bitter when fire and air predominate, such as garlic, ginger, pepper. It can also be salty when water and fire predominate; acrid when water and air predominate, such as with musk or gentian; and, finally, astringent when earth and air predominate, as with the example of myrobolan[36], the stem and fruit of which are used to heal a great number of illnesses.

In the southern temperate regions of Tibet there are numerous dense forests. Medicinal plants are rare there because, for the most part, they are eaten by wild animals. Their properties are also weaker. By contrast, in the high mountains where the summits are covered in snow and where a glacial wind whips the slopes, the plants contain substances that are rich and different from all the others. Here the rocky zones are rich in gold, silver, copper, iron, lead. In the lower-altitude regions heat plays an essential role, conferring particular substances on the medicinal plants. On these slopes stones such as turquoise can be found. Plants differ also by the direction in which they grow: turned toward the north they have a cooling effect, toward the south more of a warming effect. In Tibetan medicine a single ingredient does not suffice to bring the hoped-for cure; a combination of several ingredients is always used.

We were in the month of May. Dawn had broken and the sun was beginning to rise in a limpid sky. In the temple Khenrab Norbu had assembled a group of seven students, of which I was one. We were placed under the guidance of a *mennien*, a physician responsible for medications. This master explained to us our first mission on the snowy summits. With him we invoked the deities so that they would protect us during the ascent and assist us in finding a rare flower, of which Men-Tsee-Khang had the most urgent need. It grew only during the second, third and fourth months of the year, and a large quantity of it was necessary to produce a small amount of medicine. The prayers lasted scarcely twenty minutes. We changed our monastic robes for *chupas* and set out. The only things we brought with us were a little *tsampa* and a blanket.

We made slow progress. For three hours we beat a path through a thick forest and tried to follow the trail of a bear that seemed to have passed by there a short time before us. Zigzagging between branches torn out by a storm, we crossed numerous copses, then finally emerged from the forest and had to walk another two hours. At an altitude of almost four thousand meters, we stopped in a vale that appeared to be suspended between two peaks. At a sacred site we conducted ancestral rituals by burning a few juniper branches[37] and incense. Nearby some poles had been planted from which prayer flags fluttered in the wind. We added our own flags to them, shared our meager meal, and started out again. The vegetation gave way to a thick layer of snow, which slowed us down even more. The sun played on the mountain peaks as the day slowly declined. The air became more and more glacial, and the cold penetrated to our bones. We still had two more hours of walking. In this infinite space the physical trial sharpened our senses. The blood beat in our temples, breathing became more and more difficult. I developed a painful headache and was fearful of becoming a victim of mountain sickness at any moment.

Suddenly, on a summit dazzling with light, a convent detached itself from the rocky mass. This was Gargompa, a monastery inhabited by nuns. The welcome they gave us was warm. As soon as we arrived, they served us tea and soup, for which we felt the greatest need. Evening was falling now on the mountain and it was very cold. The eldest of the nuns gave each of us a thin mattress and a blanket that we unrolled over our *chupas*. Meditations, brief words exchanged, tired faces, heavy legs, we were finally able to stretch out, the eight of us aligned like the layers of an onion. It was then that one of our companions, Yeche Dakpa, had the formidable idea of rolling himself up in the mattress. It was funny to see and we laughed loudly and immediately did the same with more bursts of laughter. The next day Yeche Dakpa had a new name: 'the wearer of the nuns' mattress'. On the way back we picked nettles that were of much better quality than those found today in India.

In the month of May I took part in another mission, to a place called Joung-mi-ri-teu, situated at a very high altitude. The experience was rather painful because we had to stay there a full week. To fight against altitude sickness, we ate dried turnips and nettle leaves. This time there were about twenty of us, divided into groups of five or six. Early in the morning each team would head in a certain direction and would not return until nightfall. Our objective was to gather another rare plant, excellent for cardiac disease. The difficulty consisted above all of finding the precise place where this plant grew. Often students would return empty-handed, and when that happened to me, I returned to the monastery disappointed and a little ashamed. The *mennien* who accompanied us made only this comment on the little success we had: 'You'd think you'd been sleeping up there!'

A little later in the season Khenrab Norbu asked me to go with seven other students to Ei-tso. This expedition was particularly dangerous and required a physical condition able to withstand any hardship, which is why the master chose the most robust among us and never the youngest. To reach this spot, it was necessary to cross several passes and go up very high into the mountains, to the eternally snowy summits. We met some nomads who gave us shelter during the harvesting. At Ei-tso we found a medicinal plant, called *upel*, which grew in the snow. Braving the glacial cold and the dampness, we also endured great eye pain. This felt as though fine sand had been thrown into our eyes. It happened to me and my companions and rendered us almost blind for an entire day, but nevertheless we had to carry out this precious mission. Sometimes, when the pain would not stop, a dull anguish, shared by all of us, would grip me. I was afraid of losing my sight! In the evening, sheltered from the wind that was blowing in heavy gusts, in spite of everything I made the effort to learn some extracts from the *Gyushi*. Reading in the feeble light of the lamps caused me great pain, and I would see mirages surge up, changing with the different colors of the rainbow. Later I learned from medical treatises that this type of altitude sickness could be prevented. All you had to do was apply on the eyes the bile of the *kia-ka*[38], a bird well-known in our regions. Unfortunately, we did not have any at that time. It was also particularly difficult to light a fire. We were not lacking for the leaves and branches of bushes, which also served to prepare incense, but everything here proved to be very damp. The snowfalls were abundant, and it was a rare evening when we could make ourselves a little warm tea. When we had gathered enough dry firewood, and the weather permitted, we would choose a place a little removed from the nomads' camp and play a game of dice. But as always I spent most of my leisure time studying. When it was impossible to light a fire, I would hold little sticks of burning incense as close as I could to the page to decipher a few words. In spite of all the obstacles that arose before us all, I pursued my work cheerfully. I liked particularly the study of pharmacology, and I understood that the harvesting of plants was an integral part of my training to be an *amchi*.

Returning to Lhasa, I spent a little more than a month at Men-Tsee-Khang following new teachings from my master, the Venerable Khenrab Norbu, and seeing the lama who was initiating me into grammar and poetry. Then I set out again on a mission. It was the end of October. The place to which our expedition was heading was called Ma-ri-koung. There we were to pick *chou-tak*[39], the roots of which grow tangled in water and mud. Its flowers, which gave off a strong sweet perfume, were blue or white, and fine lines ran on the leaves to form patterns. Certain plants that were the most sought-after had nine nodes; others only five, six, or seven. The delicate operation of picking these plants took place ideally at the moment when the water began to freeze. Having trekked through a pass, we approached a stream. Further along was a lake, a veritable turquoise jewel. When the weather permitted, we arrived at the site rather early to look for a plant that resembled a potato.[40] An oppressive atmosphere was given off by the narrow hollow. This was a place that was not hospitable to humans.

The students responsible for the meals served us a soup called *toukpa-baktouk* that contained pellets of dough and a little meat. Every noon, I swallowed mine in silence, and would leave my companions to climb to the top of a small waterfall better to observe the blocks of ice that fell into the lake with a dull sound and created a profusion of little waves. This place had a great effect on me. Was it the cold or the atmosphere that made me tremble? Doubtless both. When I rejoined the other students, it was time to begin the gathering. We would sometimes stay whole hours in the water. We had real trouble pulling the plants out by the roots. Our legs burned, our hands were blue. I do not know how the Indians at Dharamsala do it, but they bring us some plants of excellent quality that they collect near Manali or Rewalsar.

In 1943, the year sheep-water of our calendar, I was twenty-one years old – and I was finally at the point of realizing what had been my dearest wish: under the eyes of my master, the Venerable Khenrab Norbu, and my professors, I passed the tests with brilliance. It was customary for the students of Men-Tsee-Khang to offer tea on two occasions: at the moment of their admission and after their success in the examinations on the first three volumes of the *Gyushi*. Generally the expenses for these occasions were taken care of by our home monastery. I had assumed all the expenses for my entry by borrowing from Pessala; but I was unable to face new expenses, and there was no question of borrowing again. I had written to the abbot of Chothey and to my tutor, but had received no response. I shared my embarrassment with Khenrab Norbu. The very next morning my master went to the *Kashag*, to whose members he explained my situation. A letter addressed to the Chothey monastery was prepared by Men-Tsee-Khang and approved by the members of the governing body in the course of a meeting. A few weeks later, an emissary arrived from Chothey with an envelope containing the amount needed for the ceremony. All my wishes had been fulfilled. But, with the exception of the message confided to the donkey-drivers encountered on the road to Lhasa, I had never sent any news to my tutor. I acknowledge that I was a little negligent with respect to the abbot of Chothey and my uncle-tutor, but I was absorbed by my studies.

8

The Purification of Mercury and Other Medicinal Plants

During my stay at Men-Tsee-Khang, I participated in numerous plant-gathering expeditions. In the course of two I took examinations, first as a student, then as a *mendzine*. Every two years in summer professors and students would go to the foot of a mountain situated near Lhasa to collect plants. Preparations for this expedition went on for about ten days beforehand. Tents, clothing, blankets, food, and kitchen materials were assembled. About forty of us from Men-Tsee-Khang participated, and about sixty workers, *wou-lak*, joined us for the occasion. Half of them came from a place called Do-de-Pou and the other half from Dak-yepa. The first group was led by our *mennien*; the second by a *mendzine*. The *mendzine*, who is not a doctor, is responsible for the medicines, and the *mennien*, who is a doctor, supervises them. Together they determine the right time for the harvests, supervise the plant gatherings, prepare the pills and manage the stocks of medicines. These vast campaigns entailed considerable expense, which generally assumed by the students. Nomads loaned forty to fifty yaks to transport the numerous pieces of baggage – two students shared a bag. Two of us were responsible for setting up the tents; two others took charge of the supplies.

At daybreak on the morning of the departure Khenrab Norbu called the students together in the great hall to recite prayers and invoke the favors of the deities. This ceremony lasted about twenty minutes. Then, with an indescribable hubbub, we started out. The professors led the way on horseback; the others followed on foot. The yaks slowed us down a good deal, and it took several hours to reach Do-de-Pou. As soon as we reached it, we were convened in the temple. Khenrab Norbu was seated cross-legged on a stone throne. One of our tutors was charged with reading the charter of Dessi Rinpoche, the regent who had governed the affairs of the country during the minority of the fifth Dalai Lama, and with reminding us of the basic rules to be observed for the gathering of the plants, especially for those of us assigned to collect certain plants on the northern slopes where it was colder. We were cautioned to choose the healthiest possible sites; to take the medicinal plants at the most propitious moment, fresh and not faded, although certain ones had to be picked when they were very old; to wash them carefully, then to dry them in suitable places. We were also reminded that the plants should not be kept more than three years[41] because after that they lose their medicinal properties.

Working in small groups, we spent three or four days in each zone indicated by our professors, doing strenuous work interspersed by the trumpet calls that announced meals, breaks and the end of work at nightfall. When we completed one area, we climbed about a

113

hundred meters up the mountain to another, carrying our heavy loads.

At the end of a week we arrived at a place called Yak-go-la, a pass that had the form of a yak's head. Until then the elders taught the younger ones how to find the plants and how to select them. Once we were on a site, each had to make out as best he could. At Yak-go-la we were joined by the groups that were working on another side of the mountain. They were proceeding in the same way.

In the evening we burned incense, and the youngest ones interpreted an opera from our folklore. I did not like to take part in this activity because I could not sing in tune, but the others willingly volunteered. As soon as we were in sight of the pass, they let out strange animal cries. During the festivities, two students came out of the group in turn and offered tea and *khapse*, which is a soup, to everyone. We were also responsible for the morning meal and lunch for the *wou-laks*, tradition requiring that dinner be offered them by the professors and the tutors.

When the tents had been dismantled and all the equipment assembled, we crossed the pass very early in the morning to go to another picturesque place covered with meadows and fields, called Lo-nak-tse-ka by the ancients. While the *wou-laks* set up the camp, we went to gather plants. At sunset everyone took his place according to rank and friendship. But whether it was during work or rest, we had to keep watch to separate the Do-de *wou-laks* from the Dak-yepa *wou-laks*, because they did not get along at all. It was like this with every expedition, to the point that their tents were placed at a respectful distance from each other. It was even said that in previous years fights had broken out and some of the workers had killed each other.

The *wou-laks* slept little and spent their nights singing and dancing around an immense fire. Tall spirals of smoke rose and gave off a strong smell of juniper. The singers' voices carried far, and seated alone on a rock I listened to them with immense pleasure. Sometimes wild animals approached, attracted by the noise and the smell of the soup. One day in the mountains, I had noticed some wolves who were following us. Eagles nested on the rocky peaks, and vultures circled in the sky. Snow leopards waited for their moment, when the chamois, the deer or the antelope drew near to drink from the lakes that were innumerable in this region.

Frequently a storm burst and this sudden interruption captivated me. I loved to listen to the noise of the rain and the rumble of the thunder, then the terrible cracking of the lightning on the snowy summits, suddenly illuminated. According to the strength of the storm, torrents of water engulfed the camp site, drowning the fires, drenching the men and frightening the horses and the yaks. Nervousness overtook everyone, while in the suspended twilight the roaring of the storm redoubled. The violent wind carried heavy clouds swollen with rain. The nearby lake was shaken with swirls and eddies and reverberated with the sounds of the storm. The cold intensified. In silence we huddled against each other. I would close my eyes, and when the storm was abating, I continued to listen to the singing of the rain. I smiled and allowed my memory to carry me back to the house, to the hill down which I had slid into icy water, and then to *Mola* who was watching me.

At daybreak if the bad weather persisted, we would

invoke the deities to solicit their protection. But as soon as calm was restored, we would happily set off again to pick the plants that we slipped into our *ga*, which was a type of leather sack used by nomads. At Lo-nak-tse-ka there was good visibility because the terrain was flat and our professors could observe us at work. Only once did I not succeed in gathering a sufficient number of plants. In the camp, in front of everyone, one of the professors made a remark about it. I was terribly annoyed, and it never happened again.

Every day the plants were sorted, washed, cleaned and immediately sent by yaks to Men-Tsee-Khang. To avoid any risk of a brawl, the *wou-laks* from Do-de would leave for Lhasa with the latest harvests. These expeditions always ended at Dak-yepa. We set up camp near the monastery.

The moment was important because it was here that Khenrab Norbu, surrounded by our professors and tutors, tested our knowledge of the medicinal plants. An immense tent that was held up in its center by a wooden pole had been carefully erected before our arrival. A large rectangular enclosure had been marked off around it with three openings, left, right, and center.

The test was much anticipated by the students but also by the surrounding monasteries and the aristocrats of the capital. Many people arrived at Dak-yepa to take part in the memorable day. From sunrise they would crowd in around the enclosure. After the morning prayers Khenrab Norbu installed himself in the center of three thrones set up in the front area of the tent. On his left was the oldest professor; on his right the youngest. Placed a meter in front of them were samples of the plants. Acording to the variety and abundance of the harvests, there could be several dozen.

The tests began around six o'clock in the morning. In a firm voice the *mendzine* called the students one by one. Entering the enclosure on the right, the first advanced with hesitation, bowing before the masters and placing himself to the right of the plants. On a sign from Khenrab Norbu, he had to identify the plants that were presented to him and explain their characteristics. When he had finished, another student presented himself, and so on. Sometimes one of us invented new names. I remember, for example, a plant that had the form of a rat. Not succeeding in identifying it, someone simply called it 'rat cadaver'. The observers burst out laughing, but not our professors, who did not appreciate the humorous reaction of some of us and the ignorance of others.

A proctor noted all the responses. When a student spoke in too weak a voice or showed little assurance, he was automatically called to order. At the end of the test we went out on the left and had to keep away from the other students, even in the camp that evening. A *mennien* watched us vigilantly. Our results were announced before we passed through the enclosure. When my turn came, the secretary shouted in a thundering voice:

'Tenzin Choedrak, *tik-chik tang kour-guie,*' meaning 'one wrong response and eight half-wrong responses'.

This method of tabulating the unsatisfactory responses was called in Tibetan '*tik-tsi-kour tsi*', which means the 'calculation of what is wrong and half-wrong'. *Tik* means wrong answer; the proctor represents this sign by he symbol 'O'. *Kour* means half-wrong answer, and is represented by an 'X'. *Chik* is one, and *guie* is eight. When we identified a plant but were mistaken in our explanations of the characteristics or they were not satisfactory, we were given a *kour*. So the examiners announced only *tik* and *kour*, without giving us the least information about our mistakes.

This went on for three days. On the last day everyone was assembled again for a final session. The time had come to explain the wrong answers; the correct ones were never commented on. In turn we passed before Khenrab Norbu and his assistants. At that moment you could see all the students nervously fingering their *malas*; in fact, they were using these prayer beads to make the final count of their test.

The students especially feared this session. Sometimes the youngest were more successful than the older ones. The latter were then obliged to prostrate themselves before them and cede them their places at the head of the line, because we were placed in the order of our success. Then we read the charter of Dessi Rinpoche. The first among us was honored with a prize: a block of tea in leaves, a copy of the *Gyushi* (the *Four Basic Tantras*), five pieces of brocade to wrap the sacred texts and a *kata*, the silk scarf that is presented as a sign of respect. The four runners-up were also rewarded. As for the five in last place, they had to perform a play before an amused audience. The fifth-place student played the role of a government official for medicinal plants, the fourth was a sort of innkeeper, the third was a donkey-herder, the next-to-last played the 'white donkey', and the one in last place, the 'black donkey'. Of the last two, one wore a white *chupa*, the other a black one, and both had little bells around their necks.

To the cries and jeers of the spectators they had to get down on all fours like real donkeys. In my first year at Men-Tsee-Khang I was in next to last place and had to play the 'white donkey'. The role of the 'black donkey' was considered unlucky; it was said that the romances of the students who found themselves in this role would come to nothing.

After we returned from Dak-yepa life continued as before. Several times a year I led students to gather plants on a hill near Lhasa, not far from Men-Tsee-Khang. Instead of coming directly back from these expeditions, we would take a road that passed by a field near Norbou Lingka. There we dug a long narrow ditch. The game consisted of jumping over it. We took a running start and then had to leap from a spot we had marked on the ground. We divided ourselves into two groups, the older ones and the younger, and we made bets, usually of two *khel*, about twenty-eight kilos of grain, which the losers had to pay the winner. We carried the sacks of grain to a nearby military camp where one of our companions lived. He would keep the precious booty until the new year, when we would be able to supplement our meals for the traditional *Lossar* ceremonies with this *tsampa* we had won from our games.

For *Lossar* we were authorized to leave Men-Tsee-Khang from morning to about three o'clock in the afternoon. Since I hardly touched beer, I often returned earlier but others would not come back until five or six o'clock. Their drunkenness was immediately noticed and the scenes were sometimes funny. They talked nonsense and, of course, did their best to conceal our escapades and crazy wagers. We would challenge other schools in Lhasa to test which was the most intrepid. There were about twenty schools, among them Takhang, Niarong, Kounguiour and Gokhangsar. The school of Tse was the most famous and prestigious of all and had about twenty students. But Men-Tsee-Khang was the largest, with about sixty students, all robust and courageous. The mountain air and the plant harvesting gave us muscles and broad shoulders, and also a few of the students had come from the army. Thus our stone-throwing battles were quite unequal. As soon as our professors got wind of one of our scuffles, we were punished. The chastisement for engaging in violent behaviour could be severe and we frequently paid for our misdeeds with whip lashes.

In 1944, the year monkey-wood, I became a *mendzine*. I was to remain in this position until 1952, the year dragon-water. A student who worked conscientiously was given responsibilities. There were three of us, with a heavy workload. Together we developed a year's program. If we participated in the ceremonies and the reading of texts in the morning, we were relieved of classes. We rejoined our companions for dinner and the evening prayers.

We took our turns going up the mountain. The *Khashag* would provide a letter of recommendation for recruitment of *wou-laks*. When the plants had been collected and transported to Men-Tsee-Khang, we presented them to a professor who inspected them and gave his approval for the grinding of the plants and production of the medicines. The key to the storeroom door was entrusted to one of the three of us, depending on our other jobs at the time.

In all our activities, from the plant harvesting to the preparation of the medicines, we were expected to work in a state of consciousness as close as possible to the spirit of enlightenment, and to exert ourselves to act as if we ourselves were the Medicine Buddha. The state of mind in which we accomplished these activities was said to influence favorably or unfavorably the efficacy of a remedy. When we collected the plants we were of course supposed to be aware of the sunshine, the topography, and the soil conditions, because all these elements played a part in the quality of the flowers, roots and fruit of the plants. In addition, by the clarity of our minds and the purity of our intentions we would be more, or less, apt to prepare the medicines correctly. The objective was necessary to try to attain the qualities of the Buddha, which are as vast as space. What happiness then to be able to practice them, if only for an instant! It is true, and we never forget it, that our motivation, good or bad, determines the quality of our actions. If our spiritual practice is contaminated by self-love, our capacity to accomplish good will suffer and we can never be considered good *amchis*. If I became a *Lhamenpa*, if I did not die in prison, and if I could endure, sometimes with serenity, all the sufferings that have been inflicted on me, I think it is because throughout my existence I have tried to put into practice the teachings of Buddha as much as I was able.

A good *mendzine*, this is what I also tried to become. In fact, the preparation of the medicines put our medical knowledge in contact with our spiritual disposition. All the operations of pulverizing and mixing the substances began with prayers. The spirit purified, we could then act. Once the process of transformation of the medicinal substances was begun, it could not be interrupted, no matter how long its duration, which could sometimes be several days. Certain plants had to be prepared on the spot in the mountains. We acted in conformity with the directions of the *Gyushi*: collect the herbs and clean them of minuscule grains of sand, boil them with a high flame, filter the preparation with the tail of an animal, collect the residual juice and filter it once again into a pot. Heat it, stirring it constantly, until a dark thick paste forms. It was a little like making molasses candy. From an enormous quantity of plants, only a very small amount of medicine would be obtained.

At Men-Tsee-Khang the preparation of medicines took even longer. The most robust among the young students spent hours crushing the plants into a powder which during the night was then shaped into round pills. We succeeded in fabricating about ten kilos each of two types of pills. Because they were fashioned by hand the size of the pills would vary. It would take far too long to explain in detail the transformation of the plants into medicine because we almost always used numerous ingredients. To illustrate this, take the example of a medicine that is composed of these ingredients: *routa*, *kiourou*, *bachaka*, *sindou*, *soungmi* and *pipiling*. *Routa*'s nature is cold. *Kiourou* is still colder, and *bachaka* is the coldest of the three; these three ingredients are called *sil-soum*, literally 'the three cool ones'. They have a cooling, refreshing effect on the body. The three other ingredients, *sindou*, *soungmi* and *pipiling*, have a warm nature and generally provoke body heat. Thus when one suffers from gastritis the upper part of the body becomes warm, while the lower part becomes cool. The conjunction of these two extremes causes gas to accumulate in the stomach. The sick person is then taken with vomiting and the temperature rises. The recommended medicine for this type of trouble is the *routa doupka*, 'having six *routas*', which will balance the extreme temperatures and improve the patient's condition.

Why this example? At a scientific meeting in South Korea eminent specialists touched on the problem of gastritis. I had not been invited to take part in the discussions and so I wrote on a brochure all the characteristics of this medicine, its composition and its therapeutic virtues, and I tacked it on a board at the entrance to the hall. Later I offered this document to His Holiness the Dalai Lama. Here is what I indicated: *routa* eliminates trouble associated with the 'wind' element, blood poisoning and other blood problems, as well as gas in the stomach; *kiourou* lowers fever in the blood and bile; *sindou* treats all illnesses of the stomach; *bachaka* lowers the temperature of the blood; *soungmi* contributes to curing illnesses of the kidneys and those caused by cold (low body temperature); *pipiling* treats infections of the stomach and liver, as well as illnesses caused by cold.

Supported by Australian and Korean specialists, I then had to present my approach to the problem before a large audience. I said:

'One may explain separately the specificities of each ingredient or consider the pill in its totality. If a fever is detected when a patient's pulse is taken, a medicine with an elevated proportion of the three ingredients: *routa*, *kiourou* and *bachaka* should be prescribed to lower the temperature. But if the patient's temperature is low, ingredients that produce heat, *soungmi*, *sindou* and *pipiling*, are called for. In a hundred patients suffering from gastritis, each is a unique case requiring its own special treatment.' My talk was published. It was one of my greatest hopes that it would permit a better understanding of our medical knowledge.

Let us come back to Men-Tsee-Khang. In 1950, the year tiger-iron, I was selected to go to P'ari to study a special text, a commentary on the manner of using mercury. A *tulku* by the name of Docha possessed the text and had undertaken research in this area. Docha's interest had been awakened during one of his stays in Darjeeling, where he met a German scientist who spoke to him of the medical uses of mercury. On his return to P'ari the *tulku* heard that Tibetan medicine also employs mercury and he looked for documentary evidence and found this text.

During the last two years that I was a *mendzine* I participated in the production of our famous 'precious pills', like the *rin-chen ratna sampel*, which means the 'precious jewel that crowns all hopes'. This pill is an antidote for all types of poisonings: food, plants, insect bites, animals, and chemical products. It also minimizes the toxic effects of prolonged exposure to the sun. It has a beneficial effect in the treatment of hemiphlegia, paralysis, rigidity or contractions of the limbs and the muscles, paralysis or dislocation of the joints, numerous nervous troubles that include trembling and swelling, urinary incontinence, difficulties in opening and closing the eyelids, and neuralgia pain. This pill may also be used for sensory deficits, such as deafness, loss of the sense of smell and proprioceptive sensations, or loss of the control of salivation. It exercises a regulatory effect on high blood pressure and is effective for cardiac disorders, blood clots, ulcers, and cancers in their early stages. An individual in good health may take it as a general tonic.

The precious pill contains the inestimable *ngulchou tsothel*, a preparation the base of which is composed of purified mercury, sulphur, and sixteen different metals and minerals. There are seventy other ingredients, including purified gold, silver, copper, iron, and gems such as coral, turquoise, pearl, lapis lazuli, and another gem, called *si*, that is extremely rare in Tibet. To these are added substances extracted from clove, exudate of bamboo, nutmeg, chebule myrobalan, beleric myrobalan and fruits of the emblic myrobalan.

The process of purifying mercury is extremely delicate. The production of thirty kilos of mercury requires about sixty to seventy different ingredients and involves the work of sixteen people for a period of six months. The first step takes two months and consists of extracting the poison. Without entering into all the details and because this operation should be carried out only by those who know it perfectly, we can say that raw mercury imported from India is mixed with fern root and wild ginger by placing all of them together in a piece of soft musk deer leather, which is then knotted with a cord. For days this little pocket is rubbed in the palm of the hand, long enough for the vegetal mixture to release all its properties and absorb the poisons of the mercury. The leather also absorbs some of the toxins. When the ingredients are removed from the pouch, the vegetal mixture appears black, while the mercury has a brighter color and seems cleaner. After other intermediate steps, the mercury is boiled in cow urine. During this operation certain medicinal plants, and salts and metals are added. At a more advanced stage the mercury is cooked in oil and combined with sulphur powder, which itself has undergone a purification process. When they are thus combined, the toxic effects of these two mixtures diminish further and a yellow powder is produced, which is ground for a day and a half without interruption until it becomes black and extremely fine. By this time the thirty kilos of mercury have been reduced to no more than twenty-five kilos.

Another step consists of extracting the poison from the other metals, the bronze, silver, gold, iron, lead, and copper. The metals are then melted into fine sheets the thickness of a bee's wing. A plant-base mixture is applied to them and they are dried in the sun. The gold must be heated for close to fifty-eight hours at a moderate heat; if not, it will weigh scarcely more than a piece of burnt paper at the end of the operation. The process is the same for all the other metals, but they require less heating. For the silver, ten to twelve hours are needed.

The consumption of mercury that has not been properly detoxified would prove fatal. The purification of the mercury is analogous to the purification of the mind. Take for example a person whose spirit is prey to hate, desire, ignorance, or even the will to harm others. In order to be of help to others, the spirit of such a person would have to be purified, filled with compassion, love and goodness. It is exactly the same for mercury. Once purified, the mercury becomes a precious remedy which cures many troubles. Impure or poorly detoxified, it remains a deadly poison. Moreover, before giving it to our patients we doctors try it on ourselves. Badly prepared mercury provokes a weakening of the body, intense pain and loss of digestive heat; tumors could also appear. The skin takes on a bluish color. Those are symptoms indicating the presence of toxic mercury in the body. If one absorbs too much of it, the skin peels and the teeth fall out; the vision becomes blurred or is lost. The final stage of mercury poisoning is, of course, death.

In the West everyone knows the dangers of mercury and some Western scientists do not hesitate to say that Tibetan doctors are playing with fire in using it. But we rely on the texts of the *Gyushi*: purified detoxified mercury clarifies the mind and the vision; the sense of smell is heightened and one hears with great acuity. All the senses are extremely acute. We Tibetan doctors consider it the most eminent of medicinal substances. It confers considerable strength on the body, improves the functioning of the vital organs, permits longevity and fortifies the constituent elements of the body, which are the blood, fat, muscles, bones, and bone marrow. It also works on the toxic effects of radiation treatments. Mercury also plays a preventive role against spirits or maledictions that might be directed at us. We use it in such precious pills as *rin-chen drangdjor rilnak chenmo*, the 'great precious pill black cold composite', *rin-chen tsotru dashel*, the 'precious crystal of purified moon', and *rin-chen ratna sampel*, the 'precious jewel which crowns all hopes'.

It is also important to know that medicines with a mercury base are not easily degradable. Many medicines have an expiration date beyond which they become ineffective, even harmful, but these pills do not lose their curative properties. At the school of Tse there was *tsotru** from the period of the fifth Dalai Lama.

When a patient is treated with the precious pills, it is important that certain steps be followed. At bedtime take the pill out of its capsule, crush it and put the powder in a cup of warm water that has been boiled, cover the cup with clean linen and let it sit overnight. At daybreak the next day stir the substance and drink it while reciting the mantra of the Medicine Buddha. If the mixture is too cold because of the climate, add a little warm water. Then drink a cup of warm water and remain in bed, keeping warm and well covered. Engage in few activities and remain calm. For at least two days after taking the medicine avoid meat, eggs, raw vegetables and fruits, raw cereals, garlic, fried, spicy and acidic foods. Abstain also from alcohol. Avoid stress, naps during the day, sexual relations, and cold baths. Take no other medication on the same day. Except in an emergency, the precious pill should be ingested on a favorable day, such as the full or new moon.

Not long ago I participated in a conference in the United States. To prove to the physicians that the purified mercury that we use in Tibetan medicine is not toxic, I swallowed three grams of *ngulchou tsotru* in front of them and then asked them to perform tests on me. Later some of the specialists informed me that I had a high concentration of mercury in my body. I told them that in spite of this I experienced no secondary effects, such as a weakening of the sense organs or any other trouble arising from absorption of unpurified mercury. I distributed the pills to everyone who was present. I think that some of them kept them as an exotic object, a souvenir from a somewhat eccentric doctor.

9

'May I Be . . . Their Physician, Their Remedy, Their Servant'

In 1944 (the year monkey-wood) I became a *mendzine*. I had found support from my master Khenrab Norbu, and from his confidence in me, that was indispensable in following the medical and spiritual path. He was good, compassionate, and tireless in his will to share his knowledge and wisdom with his students. Never did he abuse us. The confidence I had in him became the foundation of my life. In imitation of the Buddha he invited us to align ourselves with the master-teacher and with learning. When later I had to endure much suffering in prison I often reflected on his counsel:

> *Trust not the person, but his teaching.*
> *Trust not the words, but their meaning.*
> *Trust not the relative meaning, but the ultimate meaning.*
> *Trust not ordinary conscience, but superior wisdom.*

I had passed all my exams on the three tantras but my studies were still not finished and I was not yet recognized as an *amchi*. Meanwhile I had begun to consult at Men-Tsee-Khang. After examining the patient's pulse or urine I had to establish my diagnosis and present it to the professor. If I was mistaken he would rap me on the head, in front of the patient, who would usually laugh. Before consulting on a patient, I always brought to mind the vows and requested the favors of the divinities in arming myself against negativity and obstacles that might arise. For example, I would recite *The Call to the Deities:*

> *Deities*, rishis[42]
> *Act in accord with your words*
> *Keep us from interferences . . .*

According to the *Gyushi*, whoever desires to help others and study medicine must develop to the best of his or her ability the qualities of the physician. The texts direct one to 'have intelligence', know the medical texts on health, illness and death; have a 'white spirit', which means to be filled with the desire to come to the aid of others; be armed with commitment to the physician's vows; respect the precepts of medical ethics; have grace of the body, speech and thought; be enthusiastic in all activities, love the process of caring for the sick, and be constant and persevering. Finally, one must have the knowledge of religious practices.

These are the doctor's vows: respect the words of one's teachers as if they were those of the Medicine Buddha; respect the texts; love the students and develop affection and benevolence toward the young pupils; consider the patients with compassion, as if they were your own children; be 'as a pig or a dog', meaning never experience disgust for unpleasant substances, such as pus, urine, feces, blood.

'May I Be . . . Their Physician, Their Remedy, Their Servant'

For me, being a doctor means helping living beings above all. The Tibetan word for doctor is *Menpa*. The word *men* means 'beneficial' or 'remedy', and *pa* means 'person', thus he or she who cares for and helps others. *Menpa* may also be used for any person who accomplishes something for the good of others, not necessarily on the medical level. In the past, such people were respected as paternal figures. The *menpa* is also qualified as '*Lha-Je*', a title conferred a very long time ago by one of the Tibetan kings. According to the explanation in the Tantra, the king must also show respect for the doctor. *Amchi*, the word Tibetans commonly use for doctor, is of Mongolian origin.

A doctor must be intelligent because he is destined for great responsibilities. Intelligence allows one to distinguish between what is and is not appropriate. The parable of the rabbit and the lion teaches us that a puny fragile rabbit can outwit the powerful lion by trickery. In the same way the intelligent doctor will triumph over illness by his cleverness. If he is intelligent he will succeed in identifying the illness without having to ask himself too many questions about what might be done for the patient. It is a little like the people of Belpo in Nepal, who can judge the quality of a piece of fruit by its color alone.

The doctor's moral engagement, *dam-tsik* in Tibetan, requires strict discipline. The patient should be treated as if he were one's parent. Not to observe this vow is to create immediately an obstacle between the doctor and the patient, and then the illness will be much more difficult to treat. Moreover, if the doctor does not respect this vow he runs the risk of being reborn in an inferior kingdom, possibly in the form of an animal or a ravenous spirit.

Creativity is another quality. The doctor should display ingenuity in caring for a patient, all the while respecting to the letter the laws relative to mind, speech and behavior. One must consider how each word or gesture may affect another person. It is the same for thoughts, which should also be directed toward the well-being of others. Thus the mind should be pure and clean, and the doctor should always act in a loving and compassionate manner.

One of the vows requires enthusiasm. The doctor should love his work, whether it be for his own benefit or that of others. Another necessary quality is prudence with regard to the diagnosis and his attention to his patients. If he should be friendly, he must also be able to act with extreme firmness. If his patients are uneducated or aggressive, the doctor should face them with serenity. If not, the illness may worsen. In brief, he should know how to adapt to each situation. Personally, I think it is by kindness that a doctor will have the most influence over the sick person. This is not to say that it may not be necessary to be severe and even harsh, for the final objective is to cure the patient. And finally, it is essential that the Tibetan doctor apply the teachings of the Buddha.

When one possesses these qualities one may become a good physician and only then may one receive and truly deserve the title of *amchi*. For the doctor who does not possess all of them, it is essential that he truly feel the desire to help living beings and that he try to do his best. A person who does not have all these qualities might be called a 'small' doctor. All things being equal, the person whose heart is filled with goodness will have better results than the one who is without it. For my part, then and still now, I do my best to cultivate these qualities, which admittedly can prove difficult.

A person who is grasping and aggressive, who stubbornly refuses to change his habits or attitudes, will not change his behavior even if you ask him to. He is as if covered with the dust of ignorance. He experiences no compassion. In this life, he battles to obtain personal benefit, and he turns his nose up at others. Such a person cannot correctly study medicine. He cannot become useful, nor can he be resourceful. That is why it is preferable not to give him this knowledge, because he would not respect either the physician's vows or the teachings of his professors and he would win the kingdom of hell in his following lives. The student who receives medical teachings, such as those of the *Four Tantras*, should always hold his professors in high esteem, and respect them deeply. He who is capable of applying these promises to perfection and has achieved these qualities could, if necessary, abandon his fortune and sacrifice his life.

Chantideva, the Indian Buddhist sage of the seventh century, said:

> *As long as space endures,*
> *As long as there are beings,*
> *May I remain*
> *To assuage the suffering and misery of the world*
>
> *As long as there are suffering beings,*
> *And until their illnesses are cured,*
> *May I be their physician, their remedy, their servant*

I do not know know if I possessed all the qualities required to become a good physician in the full sense of the term. In any case I did my best and tried to apply what my masters taught me. When I was first consulting in Tibet I encountered scarcely any patients who were difficult to treat. Nevertheless, those who suffered from depression posed some problems. I remember a monk of the monastery of Samding whom I visited several times. He suffered greatly and quarreled with everyone. No-one had been able to overcome his terrible illness and Khenrab Norbu asked me to take charge of the case. The first time I visited I found the monk seated on the roof of the monastery. He made no response to my greeting. I asked him to say some prayers with me, which he agreed to do. As he grew somewhat more confident, he confided in me his intention to commit suicide. In spite of my exhortations he remained determined. On my return to Men-Tsee-Khang I related all this to Khenrab Norbu. He advised me on the medicines to prescribe for the monk and I returned to see him the next day and on the following days.

The poor man continued to cause great problems and worry, refusing to take the medications I had brought him. He persisted in wanting to drown himself in the waters of the nearby lake. Finally, I persuaded him to accompany me to Men-Tsee-Khang, where he met my master, who took his pulse. At a signal the students grabbed his wrists and held him immobile for the time it took to apply moxibustion[43] to his sixth and seventh vertebrae[44] and to his chest. In the case of mental disturbances, my master inserted heated needles of gold, silver, and other metals, whose points were coated with a medicinal substance. The monk left Men-Tsee-Khang still in a highly charged emotional state. I continued to visit him for three consecutive days. Although his condition was stabilized, he kept insisting that he was sicker than before and that he was going to drown himself.

After a week, however, I noticed an improvement. He was smiling and had lost his aggressiveness. He had even recovered a certain confidence in life. The proof was when he told me that he had gone to the banks of the Kyitchou river, which ran around the capital, with the intention of ending his days, but did not have the courage to throw himself in.

'Act always in a way to do good.' I did everything possible to apply this maxim continually. Many years later when I resumed my functions with His Holiness the fourteenth Dalai Lama, I had to go to the region of Bylakouppe, one of the fifty-six Tibetan villages in the south of India. I made the acquaintance of a family that owned a valuable cow. This cow was coughing. In spite of several visits to the veterinary clinic and energetic treatments, the cow's condition was declared incurable. The sacred texts say that one must try to help all living beings, so I asked to see her and administered the precious pill *rin-chen ratna sampel*. She recovered in a few days. The cow's owner, an old Tibetan woman, spread the word to the whole village about the blue pill that cured cows. Of course, she did not know it was the precious pill. During my entire stay at Bylakouppe, poor people kept coming to ask me, not for medicines for themselves, but for some 'blue pills for the cows'.

'But who told you about that?' I asked them. A man answered me:

'It's Phunetsok over there, whose cow you cured and who has worn this pill around her neck ever since.'

A doctor owes his assistance to anyone who asks for it.

Part Two

1950–1976

10

And I Became a Lhamenpa

It was September 1949, the year oxen-earth of our calendar. Rumors were circulating in Lhasa that the Chinese army had penetrated Tibetan territory. They said Beijing no longer concealed its intentions to 'liberate' Tibet. Chinese troops were occupying the Amdo region, today called Qinghai by the Chinese, and they had seized the tenth Panchen Lama, who was then ten years old and who became a precious political hostage. Already some inhabitants of the capital willingly saluted the 'great wisdom and courage' of a certain Mao Zedong, of whom, I must admit, I had never heard. But most Tibetans were determined to fight against foreign interference. In the face of this powerful Chinese army, however, we could marshal at most only eight thousand men, about fifty artillery pieces, two hundred and fifty mortars, and two hundred machine guns. But we were not lacking courage.

With the growing threat from China, the *Kashag* decided to bring forward the ceremony of enthroning the fourteenth Dalai Lama. This took place on 17 November, 1950, in the year tiger-iron of the Tibetan calendar. Tenzin Gyatso was then sixteen years old. His first political act was to name two Prime Ministers, Lobsang Tachi, a monk, and Loukhangwa, a layperson. Because the Communist threat had become more focused, they advised Kundun to have part of the treasury, the gold powder and silver ingots, transported to Sikkim, where it was to remain in its hiding place for many years. The *Kashang* soon concluded from our country's isolation that the Dalai Lama's life had to be protected, all the more so because the Panchen Lama was already in the hands of the Communists. And so Kundun abandoned the 'city of the gods' to find refuge at Yatoung, three hundred kilometres from Lhasa, on the border of Sikkim, where he installed his provisional government.

A report reached him a short time later, signed by Ngabo Ngaouang Jigme, governor of the region of Kham. To avoid an invasion whose consequences could only be disastrous for Tibet, he was advised to negotiate with the Communists. A Tibetan delegation went to Beijing where discussion began on 29 April, 1951, the year hare-iron. A few weeks later, on 23 May, under threats and pressure the delegation signed the 'Seventeen Point Accord'. At the end of this document the Chinese authorities affixed a counterfeit of the seals of the Tibetan signatories. This accord delivered Tibet over to the Chinese and our country was henceforth to cease to exist as a sovereign nation. Powerless and deprived of allies, we could only submit to the dictates of Beijing in spite of the Tibetan government's total opposition to this falsified document.

Five months later, the inhabitants of Lhasa awoke one morning under the Chinese boot. It was 26 October, 1951. Three thousand Chinese soldiers were entering the capital. When I saw all those soldiers armed to the teeth, I knew that the Tibetans were under siege. I withdrew into the Jokhang temple and prayed to Tara. My prayer was this:

> *Homage to you who reside at the heart of a flaming garland,*
> *Like the fire at the end of a cosmic era.*
> *With your right leg extended and your left leg bent,*
> *You destroy the enemies of those who wish to turn*
> *The wheel of the Dharma.*

For the first time airplanes rumbled above our plateaus and trucks raised storms of dust. Immediately large-scale construction works began, especially those needed for communication. The Communists, who portrayed themselves as missionaries, spoke at length with the population assembled near Norbulingka. Their message was simple: 'We are here to liberate and modernize Tibet.'

They undertook a vast building program. The Chinese also distributed enormous amounts of money. Their coins must have weighed almost twenty-three grams but this money, dispensed to the Tibetans with such a show of generosity, was the fruit of the pillaging committed by the Communist army in Xining and elsewhere. Thousands of Tibetans collaborated with the occupiers. As a result of their sudden wealth some even went to India to start up businesses.

In prison and even many years later, I often reflected on this situation. People made jewelry with the money the Chinese gave them, but also ritual objects, conchs and large horns. Public opinion in Lhasa seemed more and more favorable to the occupiers. No-one had ever seen so much money, and for many this vision alone blinded them to reason. Some, however, were suspicious of this kindness and generosity, especially coming from armed men. The method was clever and fooled the world. Loudspeakers played songs in the streets. All this was so new. Everything seemed so believable.

The Communists pretended they would return home as soon as their mission was completed and we believed them. The greed of certain Tibetans was so great that they forgot to think about the consequences. Certainly the Chinese really did build schools, bridges, hospitals, and roads, and the standard of living in Tibet improved. At least for a few months.

Twenty-five thousand Chinese military were posted in Lhasa. The question of supplying them was the occasion for a rupture between the occupier and the Tibetan government. The population, lay and religious together, suffered the first extortion. The officers of the Popular Army of Liberation demanded twenty thousand tons of barley. The *Kashag* let it be known that such a quantity of grain was not available from the state's reserves. The Tibetan drama then took a drastic turn in quite a different direction. Inflation set in, foodstuffs became scarce, there were shortages for the first time in our history, and later, in 1961, famine made its appearance.

As the more realistic observers feared, the roads that had been built were used to introduce still more men and war machines into Tibet, and to evacuate the wood from our forests, our minerals, our resources. In addition our religious artworks were pillaged from the monasteries, which were being demolished systematically.

At the end of the year hare-iron and at the beginning of the year dragon-water (1952), a part of Kundun's family was in India. *Amala*[45], the Dalai Lama's mother, and the youngest of her sons, Ngari Rinpoche, were settled in India, at Kalimpong in a house rented by Tsering Dreulma, the Dalai Lama's elder sister. They were joined by another of her sons, Guielo Theundroup, and his wife, and then later by the oldest son, Thoupten Jigme Norbou, who had succeeded in fleeing from the great monastery of Koumboum, which had fallen into the hands of the Chinese. Jetsune Pema, the youngest of the daughters, was pursuing her studies in the Catholic convent school of Loreto in Darjeeling. I did not yet know any of them.

His Holiness had been staying in the Potala, where he was attentively following the evolution of the situation in Tibet and at the same time working on advanced studies of the Dharma. He received word that his mother had become gravely ill. The Dalai Lama shared his apprehensions with his entourage. *Amala* had consulted several Indian and Western doctors in India but without any improvement in her health, and she was calling for a Tibetan doctor. Kundun immediately summoned the director of Men-Tsee-Khang and ordered that his best doctor be sent to Kalimpong. Khenrab Norbu thought of me and indicated his choice to His Holiness. I was then thirty years old and had just passed my examinations and been placed first. According to tradition the person in first place is eligible to be named the Dalai Lama's personal physician. The person in second place would be appointed the doctor of an important district. The person in third place could hardly aspire to such honors. Four certificates of my appointment as physician to the Dalai Lama's mother were prepared: one for the *Kashag*, a second for Men-Tsee-Khang, a third for the district to which I belonged, and the last copy for me. Khenrab Norbu congratulated me on my promotion and let me know that it delighted him.

I was honored by such confidence, but I still anguished over this great responsibility. I kept telling myself that if the treatment succeeded, I would be covered with praise. But in the opposite case? Until the day of my departure, I spent much time with Khenrab Norbu, who lavished me with advice and behaved in ways to stimulate my self-confidence.

Our supplies and medicines had been loaded on mules and an escort was to guide me as far as Kalimpong. There would be sixteen days of travel in particularly difficult conditions. Some members of the Dalai Lama'a family accompanied me. There was also Namguiel, who managed the household, and Damdul, in charge of the mules, and the servants. The caravan left Lhasa at daybreak and headed in the direction of Dong-Tse, which we reached after a long week of walking. Chandzeu Kala, the treasurer of the Dalai Lama's family, was waiting for us and would accompany us to Kalimpong. Everything went marvelously well. The population, who felt the greatest respect for Kundun and for his family, welcomed us with much kindness and attention. As for me, the people surrounded me because in their eyes I occupied a most respectable position: *amchi* of *Amala*. They considered me a little like a divinity. As I was hardly used to being treated with so much reverence I experienced some discomfort which only added to my trouble and doubts.

And I Became a Lhamenpa

Amala was known in all Tibet for her generosity, kindness and compassion; she was venerated as a manifestation of Tara. The thought of having to care for her suffering body within a few days made me suddenly conscious of the eminent responsibility that Kundun and Khenrab Norbu had bestowed on me. The more we advanced in our trip the more nervous I became. Did I have enough knowledge? Above all did I possess the six qualities of a good physician? I was no longer sure.

In the evening, I prayed to Tara but as soon as I lay down I was assailed again by a multitude of doubts. I knew it was not healthy to allow my mind to be seized like that, for doubt generates failure. The world appreciates little those whose nature brings them to doubt. In a thousand ways doubt can surge up in one. One day the poet Milarepa went into a grotto. It was dark all around him and the obscurity caused him to think that a demon was crouching in the shadows. According to the story, at this precise moment a demon actually emerged. Intrigued, Milarepa asked him: 'Where do you come from?' 'I am born of your mind's doubt,' answered the demon.

The weather deteriorated when we reached the plains of P'ari. Our progress was considerably slowed by a storm. The wind carried heavy clouds of sand. Although the horses were in a panic, the guides did not slow the pace. We changed direction to try to circumvent this area. For three days we had not been able to set up a camp. We slept on the ground, rolled up in our *chupas* and a blanket and huddled against each other. We used our supplies for shelter. It was absolutely necessary not to unharness the horses and the mules who would otherwise have wandered off and been lost in the storm. We all had to protect each other, humans and animals alike. The nights were glacial but it was impossible to light a fire. Howling wolves prowled the plateau. Snow leopards would approach but as soon as they caught our smell they went back to their distant hiding places. We finally escaped the storm and made a long stop, to get rid of the sand, dry out, clean the horses and the mules, and finally drink some tea and eat a little dried yak meat.

Two days later we crossed the pass of Natula. In another two days we reached Sikkim, where we left the horses and mules with a trustworthy guard. Finally we arrived in Kalimpong after taking a car for part of the last leg of the journey, and a train for the other part. It was my first ride on a train and I had to laugh at its wheezing and blowing.

We had left Lhasa in September 1952. We were to remain in Kalimpong until the beginning of the next year. *Amala* lived in Pundah Cottage, a bungalow that she occupied with her family. Prostrations, exchanges of *katas*, and then *Amala* asked me to tell her about the situation in Lhasa. I explained it to her in a few words, and immediately I changed the subject to how I was going to make an assessment of her condition. As I took her pulse, she recited the mantra *Om Mani Padme Hum*, and fingered old prayer beads that she had kept from Taktser, the village in the Amdo where she was born. The illness was serious; her face was very pale and she seemed to me extremely weak. But as the days passed, her confidence grew. Her condition stabilized and I prescribed a pill called *pang-guien-15* and moxibustion.

I made a new diagnosis every day, in the morning, at noon, and in the evening. I administered her medicine, practiced moxibustion. I verified an improvement in her condition at the end of two weeks. But one morning she called for me a little earlier than usual and told me she did not feel at all well. I took her pulse but observed no particular trouble. I was surprised and she doubtless noticed a slight uneasiness in my expression. She must have been enjoying herself already. I took up her left hand again, then the right; her pulse was normal. I looked at her eyes. Suddenly she laughed.

'Maybe I just had a little too much *iha-tse* last night.' And *Amala* laughed heartily. She happily made fun of my confusion, knowing that I did not understand the Amdo dialect and so did not get the meaning of the word *iha-tse*. Finally she put an end to my anxiety by telling me she had eaten a very strong pepper.

'I assure you, *Amchila*, I feel much better. I just wanted to test your abilities and have a little joke.' This time, we both laughed. The little prank drew me to her and made me appreciate her even more. I discovered a very honest and also very pious woman. In the evening after dinner we never failed to invoke Tara in a prayer that she especially loved:

Homage to she whose diadem expands with moonlight,
And whose adornments flame.
From Amitabha, who is seated on your abundant hair,
Streams a light that cannot be tarnished.

Although *Amala*'s health was improved, she did not recover entirely. She remained quite frail and so I regularly gave her *rine-chen ratna sampel*. At Men-Tsee-Khang the rumor ran that I had cured *Amala*. How far away was the time when they had treated me as a simpleton! At *Amala*'s request I continued to visit her every day and through the weeks and the months we became fast friends.

Amala opted to return to Tibet with her eldest daughter and her daughter's husband to support His Holiness in the exercise of his new responsibilities. On our return I made a disturbing discovery. The Chinese propaganda had reached our people with full force. It was now considered good form in Lhasa to wear red scarves, the emblem of the Communists. Many Tibetans wore their hair up in the Chinese style and did not hesitate to abandon certain of our traditions, for example, by cutting their long beautiful hair.

In the year horse-wood (1954), His Holiness was invited to Beijing. For several months now the Chinese had effected a policy of terrible repression in Tibet. Their objective was to sabotage the international diplomatic efforts initiated by Kundun and the *Kashag*. China was all the more concerned about keeping the attention of the rest of the world off the situation in Tibet, because recent uprisings of the Khampas[46] tribes in the eastern part of the country risked the political and military involvement of the United States. There was also a question of the Dalai Lama's going to Washington, but alas, dissuaded by certain members of his entourage, he never undertook the trip.

Rumors of the imminent departure of Kundun for China circulated. The populace of Lhasa feared for his life and was vociferously opposed to this trip. In the course of a religious ceremony at Norbulingka he did his best to reassure us and promised to return the following year at the latest. The Dalai Lama left Lhasa on 11 July, 1954, escorted by Chinese troops commanded by General Zhang Jingwu. The banks of the Kyitchou river, which His Holiness had to cross in a small yak-skin boat, were off limits to the Tibetans for fear they would throw themselves into the water. The Dalai Lama was accompanied on this long and complicated journey by one of his personal physicians, Khen Choung, who died shortly after his return to Lhasa in 1955.

By 1955 (the year sheep-wood) China was the absolute master of Tibet. The Communist powers engineered the adoption of a new constitution as well as a 'resolution on the establishment of a preparatory commission for the Autonomous Region of Tibet', which was supposed to facilitate the absorption of the Tibetan government by the Popular Republic of China. This commission was to function as the central administration of Tibet, in place of our government. The Dalai Lama was designated its president, but he exercised no power. This was only for effect, the political line of authority having been decided by the party. When the Khampas revolted, Beijing responded with atrocities. Troops rolled into Lithang, Bathang, Dergue, Chamdo, and Kanze. The Khampas horsemen fiercely opposed them. In 1956 (the year monkey-fire), at the request of the Dalai Lama, the Communists accepted a truce but this was only a subterfuge to give them time to reorganize their men who were blockaded in the mountains. Almost immediately afterwards, the Chinese armies attacked our cities and our monasteries.

After the death of His Holiness's personal physician, a successor had to be found. The *Kashag* invited six students who had graduated with highest honors from

Men-Tsee-Khang, and lots were drawn. At the end of the ceremony two names were announced: that of Yeunten Thartchine, who was to die later in the Chinese jails, and mine. We were officially named *Lhamenpa* in 1956, a short time before His Holiness departed for Sikkim. In the Potala we met two other physicians who were much older than us, who also occupied this function. Both of them later died in prison. Today I am the only survivor of the four. This memoir is intended to honor them as well as all the others who perished.

My appointment as physician of the Dalai Lama having been confirmed, I immediately requested an audience with him. In August His Holiness received me in the great hall of Norbulingka. The moment was extremely intense for me. At the time the Dalai Lama was a young man of twenty-one, and heavy responsibilities already weighed on his shoulders. I had never met him before and I was very moved. He was our spiritual 'protector' and our 'refuge'. But I also felt an intense joy, a deep happiness, a little like the old Tibetans when they arrive these days in Dharamsala. All they wish for is to receive a benediction from His Holiness, and when they have obtained an audience, they go away happy and at peace and ready to leave this world if the hour should come.

So I arrived before Kundun. I prostrated myself three times and presented a *kata*. His Holiness signaled to me to approach and asked me some questions:

'What region are you from?'

'My family is from Nyemo.'

'Which monastery were you in?'

'Chothey.'

The Dalai Lama watched me with what I took for a

malicious expression. He wore thick glasses which he pushed up on his nose with a methodical gesture. Suddenly he burst out laughing with a resonant, loud laugh that immediately made me think of *Amala*, but I dared not tell him so. Then he questioned me on my trip to Kalimpong and his mother's condition, which greatly worried him. He asked me where I was living and whether I wanted to remain in Norbulingka. Since I still had other patients to see, living there would be rather awkward. As I withdrew from his presence my heart was beating so hard I thought it would burst.

While I feel very old now, I have known the joy of serving His Holiness the Dalai Lama and his family over the years. On the question of our fleeting happiness, Guieloua Guendune Gyatso, the second Dalai Lama, used to say:

> *Listen to the song of a happy man!*
> *Soon these illusory conditions*
> *That created all the scenes of my life*
> *Will be wiped out by themselves.*

As tradition required, immediately after the audience I went to Chang-Sep-Char*, the residence of the Yapchi family, a majestic house with about sixty rooms that looked out onto an immense garden. I bowed before *Amala* and presented her with a white silk scarf as a sign of good wishes.

The next day I saw the Dalai Lama again in my official capacity, which essentially consisted of taking his pulse and, as necessary, preparing medicines for him, the ingredients of which were identical to those administered to other patients. His Holiness enjoyed excellent health most of the time. With the exception of a few chills for which I treated him, I cannot say that he ever caused me any concern. I remember well, of course, this first pulse-taking. Kundun was looking at me, amused, and was laughing. In fact, he always laughed through the consultation.

A few days later Kundun was pleased to see me settle in at Chang-Sep-Char. He saw only advantages there for me. My visits continued and he appeared more and more curious about medicine. He questioned me on illnesses and I responded, trying to be as precise as possible. During these conversations, we never referred to the situation of our country.

At Chang-Sep-Char I occupied a room on the first floor. A servant prepared my meals but it often happened that I shared the table of the Yapchi family. *Amala* herself did the cooking and would invite everyone, including the household managers and the servants, to share her abundant food. This was very rare among the Tibetan aristocrats, who usually insisted on keeping their distance from inferiors. Ngari Rinpoche, the third grand incarnation of the family after Thoupten Jigme Norbu and Tenzin Gyatso, was still an adolescent. He often joined me in my rooms, where he begged me to tell him stories about Aku Tempa, the ones my father regaled me with so marvelously in the evenings by the hearth. His Holiness's grandmother also lived with us. On several occasions I also encountered Heinrich Harrer, the future author of *Seven Years in Tibet*. He would come to visit *Amala* and would volunteer to take care of the trees in the garden. He built a canal and a dam near the Kyitchou river and planted some shrubs along its banks.

In winter, when *Amala* or the grandmother caught cold, I prepared medicine for them and spent time chatting about pleasant things. However, they were both very worried about the Chinese presence in Tibet. I saw the grandmother only rarely. She frequently suffered from headaches and would sometimes be silent for an entire day. In the morning she prayed until eleven o'clock. She would have lunch at noon, do some embroidery or a little gardening until about four o'clock, and then go back to her room.

The Dalai Lama's grandmother often told this story, which I would listen to attentively: 'There was once a weaver who kept her child by her while she worked. One day, when she had to leave the house, a poisonous serpent entered the room. The family dog saw the reptile dangerously approaching the child, killed it and cut its head off with a furious bite. Then he went out to curl up in the summer sun. When the mother returned and saw her dog licking blood from its mouth, she thought he had attacked her child, and she struck the animal so violently that it died. She ran inside and there discovered the decapitated serpent and her child healthy and safe. The weaver wept a long time with remorse, bitterly regretting having killed her dog, who had saved her child's life.'

In November 1956 (the year monkey-fire) the Maharadja Kumar of Sikkim, president of the Buddhist society of the Indian Sub-Continent, invited the Dalai Lama and the Panchen Lama, whom I had still not met, to come to the ceremonies of Buddha-Jayanti to celebrate the 2,500th anniversary of the birth of Buddha. After endless negotiations with the Chinese officials in Lhasa,

Kundun and his close entourage received authorization to go. His Holiness asked me to remain in Lhasa, which I did. I took advantage of the time to study. It was around this time that my family learned I had become a *Lhamenpa*. When merchants arrived from Nyempo or from the region of Chothey, they sometimes brought me *tsampa* sent by my family.

11

The Day Everything Toppled

In 1959 Kundun already knew that Tibet was heading for ruin. The more our sovereign reflected on the future, the less he held out any hope of the Chinese leaving our land. I could sometimes read an infinite sadness in his face but he said nothing about it to me. He had assured his tutors that he would take his final monastic examinations at the time of the festivities of *Monlam*.

That year, more than in others, a huge crowd gathered in Lhasa. Kundun had settled at his summer residence, Norbulingka, which he preferred to the Potala. The reports that he received from the Amdo and Kham were catastrophic: the monasteries destroyed, the monks buried alive, young girls sterilized, women forced to abort. The soldiers of the Popular Army of Liberation committed the most appalling acts. Rumors surged in Lhasa and spread like wildfire: it seemed increasingly possible that the Communists would seize our sovereign. Almost everywhere placards were put up demanding the departure of the Chinese and denouncing the 'Seventeen Point Accord'.

On 5 March the Chinese supreme commander in Lhasa sent two emissaries to the Dalai Lama with an invitation to honor a theatrical presentation with his presence. A strange invitation indeed. The rumors intensified in the streets of the capital. The next day His Holiness brilliantly passed his last examination for the degree of master of metaphysics. The crowd continued to assemble noisily around the summer residence. They wanted to prevent Kundun from attending this presentation which had been organized by the occupiers. It all smelled of a trap.

What the Tibetans did not yet realize was that Lhasa and its surroundings had become an immense construction site. In the streets, the parks and the gardens, the Chinese had dug trenches, filled with sacks of sand and disguised by enormous blocks of wood. The city was in fact under siege by an army ready at any moment for combat. The citizens of Lhasa had seen so many strange things since the Communists occupied the city that they were not made too uneasy by these preparations.

Fearing demonstrations by the crowds at the festivities of *Monlam*, the authorities had posted heavily armed men. On the other side of the Kyitchou river, now forbidden to the populace, there was much activity in the military camp, and on the neighboring hills, cannons and mortars were now trained on the Potala, Norbulingka, and the other nerve points of the capital. This explained perhaps the absence of Chinese soldiers in the center of the city.

To sow even more confusion in people's minds, the army forced some Tibetans to disguise themselves as Khampa resisters and made them break into houses at night to rob the inhabitants of their grain and possessions. In the course of the break-ins, the women and girls of the household were systematically raped and brutalized. The objective of these barbarous acts was to spread confusion among the population and discredit the Khampas, who were the only ones who opposed the Chinese with a guerilla army in the mountains surrounding the capital.

On the morning of 10 March, I was part of the crowd, a few steps from Norbulingka. I noticed a mob of women at Drebou Lingka, venting their anger and shouting slogans: 'Chinese, out of Tibet!' 'Give us back our freedom!' 'Stop the plot against Gyalwa Rinpoche!' I did not quite realize what was happening, but I cannot have been the only one. The crowd grew as the minutes went by. More and more of the women were shouting their hatred of the occupiers. Through loudspeakers, the Chinese issued warnings and ordered the populace to disperse. The confusion was total and I admit that I was afraid. Curiously, the Chinese had hung effigies that were supposed to represent American women, probably as symbols of capitalism, on poles all over Lhasa. Now men in the crowds of Tibetans were tearing them down. Tension continued to mount. In front of the Dalai Lama's summer residence the crowd became more threatening. Framed by Chinese guards, a Tibetan minister, Tsewang Rine-dzine, prepared to enter Norbulingka. He never reached the door. The frenzied crowd started throwing stones at him and the rumor flew that he was a well-paid spy of the Chinese. As far as I knew, this man was on excellent terms with our sovereign, but how to explain that to this unleashed mob on the verge of a riot? Hatred for the Chinese was such that if you even suggested that your neighbor was friendly to the occupiers, the person would be beaten immediately. Everywhere suspicion had slyly insinuated itself, even within the Dalai Lama's immediate entourage.

The rumor was also spreading that His Holiness, accompanied by his cabinet, would finally attend the theatrical presentation organized by the Chinese. This was incomprehensible to the people of Lhasa. Ten, twenty, thirty thousand people, in a state of excitement now out of control, spontaneously moved to lay siege to the entrances of the summer residence to prevent the Dalai Lama from going into the Communist camp. The crowd seized other members of the government who were in a Jeep under Chinese escort. The passage to Norbulingka was now completely blocked. A man appeared at the main door bearing a message from the *Kashag* telling everyone to calm down immediately. A serious incident now occurred right under my eyes. A man dressed as a Chinese and armed with a pistol was riding a bicycle in the direction of Norbulingka. It was Pakpala Kentchoung who was known for his dealings with the Communists. The crowd turned on him and stoned him to death.

I finally succeeded in getting inside Norbulingka to join the representatives of the different social groups of Tibet. In my role as *Lhamenpa*, I occupied the fifth rank in the Tibetan hierarchy, which conferred on me a certain authority. The objective of the assembly was to discuss the conditions of a negotiation with the Chinese. Seven or eight groups met with the *Kashag* in the garden at the entrance to Shab-Ten-Khang, one of the largest halls of the residence. It was essential to know who was loyal and who could not be trusted. So the first order of business was to make lists of names to distinguish the 'rice eaters' from the '*tsampa* eaters'. The Tibetan administration itself was giving in to pressure from the occupiers and certain ministers were veritable puppets in their pay. The second point concerned the measures to be taken to resolve our problems with the Chinese: we were all in agreement that the military opposition was impossible since our forces were almost non-existent in the face of the Popular Army of Liberation. We knew also that a return to violence would provoke massacres of the populace. We took a break toward noon and then continued the discussions around three o'clock. This time they were held inside the hall. Everyone again gave his opinion.

We were so naive. In fact we had no proposal to present to the Chinese authorities. The peaceful solution was not the one chosen by the occupiers. Several functionaries were pressing the cause of the Communists but their behaviour was not surprising. They had grown fat and rich these last few years. It was deplorable and cowardly. A man by the name of Aga, who was a representative of Ganden monastery, called for the most extreme prudence. As an important person in the monastery he enjoyed considerable influence in the Tibetan community, but everyone was also aware of his allegiance to the Chinese from whom he had received large sums of money. He was not the only one to hold himself apart from the discussions. I did not see him but they said that a man by the name of Cheinse, who had kept silent during the debates, jumped on a motorbike and fled. These people were only puppets, bound hand and foot to our occupiers. A saying had it that these people 'kept their stomachs inside, but turned their mouths outward'. In my eyes they were traitors.

Meanwhile the Chinese patrolled the city in Jeeps shouting messages of appeasement and enjoining the crowds to return home. The Tibetans who were mouthpieces of the Communists were also encouraging the masses to remain peaceful. Violent opposition would have been useless in any case. The troops had manned the trenches and deployed their mortars and cannons. The city was surrounded by several thousand soldiers.

Kundun was also opposed to violence. On 10 March, at around one o'clock in the afternoon, he despatched three ministers to General Tan Kuan-sen to explain the situation and inform him of his refusal of the invitation. Later in the afternoon His Holiness made a strong address to the populace of Lhasa, imploring them not to give in to force or respond to provocation. The Dalai Lama promised to do everything through negotiation to resolve the question of the occupation, and he noted that China and Tibet in the past had concluded several peace accords and treaties recognizing their respective sovereignty. One of the first dated back to the eighth century, when three pillars commemorating a treaty had been erected: one before the temple of Jokhang, the second at Goungar Merou on the Sino-Tibetan border, and the third in Chang An, the Chinese capital of the time. Moreover, after chasing the Nationalist Chinese out of Lhasa in 1913, the thirteenth Dalai Lama had reconfirmed our country's independence: 'We are a modest, religious, and independent nation,' he had declared.

It is certain that Tibet was an independent state with its own customs, its own language and literature. Would you like a small example of what differentiates us from the Chinese Communists? The Tibetans love to wear rather imposing earrings; but it would never occur to the Chinese to adorn themselves this way. No, there was no resemblance between us and them. We had our own currency, our own army, our flag. Everything was there to prove that Tibet was a free and independent nation, at least until 1950.

This tenth of March, 1959, which later became the day of our national commemoration, marked my last meeting with Kundun for many years. In other times these meetings brought thirty to three hundred people together, and in the course of the hour we would discuss nominations, His Holiness's audiences, and the social and political situation of our country. On this day there were only a few of us with our sovereign and our words were quite different.

Soon we heard the first cannon fire on Lhasa.

At nightfall I was able to reach Chang-Sep-Char, where I found the Dalai Lama's grandmother and a few other members of his entourage. *Amala*, his mother, remained with him at Norbulingka. The next day, 11 March, I received a message from him setting a meeting for 14 March at the summer residence. This was the order I had been waiting for to go to Norbulingka. It was necessary that we change nothing in our habits under risk of raising the suspicions of the Chinese and their henchmen. I remained at Chang-Sep-Char with the grandmother, some members of his close entourage and the servants. Our plan was that after 14 March we would attempt to reach neighboring India. As *Lhamenpa*, my place was at the side of His Holiness.

During the night of 11 or 12 March, I was awakened by cannon fire. The sky was raked with light and there was shouting. We were afraid. The Chinese military had moved to the offensive. Their first targets were the Potala and Norbulingka. I grabbed my *mala*, the prayer beads that His Holiness had blessed, ran down the stairs, and dashed to the room of Kundun's grandmother. There was no-one. The servants had carried her to the cellar, where she was joined by the rest of the household. I was the last to arrive. We all prayed for the Dalai Lama's safety.

None of us had ever experienced a bombing. A hill concealed the rest of the city from our view so that we could not completely see what was happening. The mortar shells were crashing down on Norbulingka, the Potala, and Chagpori. I can still picture our poor guards dressed in their bright red *chupas* and armed with simple rifles or swords. They were just so many living targets for the Chinese soldiers, who were outfitted in their sand-coloured camouflage uniforms. I took a chance going into the garden, climbed the little wall and saw men, women and children fleeing. The racket from the weapons almost obliterated their cries and shouts. Chagpori was destroyed. Houses were in flames. The horror had certainly begun in 1949, when the Chinese invaded our country, but we had kept alive a feeble hope. That night, however, I understood that Tibet had ceased to exist. I wept and I prayed to Tara before rejoining the others in the cellar.

At daybreak Chang-Sep-Char was bombed in turn. The first shell fell in the garden, followed by a second, and a third, and then an incessant rain of projectiles beat down on us and on the dwelling of the Yapchi family. The palisades were battered. The windows exploded. We had twenty-five monk-soldiers to defend us. I took the hand of the grandmother, who was weeping and murmuring: *Om Mani Padme Hum.* I repeated the mantra with her several times.

We heard spurts of machine-gun fire, the barking of orders, and then repeated blows on the cellar door, which suddenly shattered. Little men wearing the red star surged in. They were all young, armed to the teeth, with ferocious faces and hateful expressions. They signaled to us to raise our hands high above our heads. They broke everything that was still intact and searched us to see if anything was being concealed. The least movement and we would have been dead! There were children among us, some of them wounded. The soldiers pointed their bayonets and pushed us toward the exit. I saw then that Chang-Sep-Char, that beautiful building, had been mostly destroyed.

I felt great anxiety for Kundun as we were being bound hand and foot. His Holiness, with his mother, his brother, Lobsang Samden, and the rest of the family, were surrounded in Norbulingka. Had they perhaps been able to flee? Were they alive? I did not know.

Because of her advanced age, the Dalai Lama's grandmother was released, which greatly relieved me. The rest of us were ordered to walk in single file to the house of the Tsarong family, where I was to be held for three weeks. I found there inhabitants of Lhasa and of Shol, many of them young people who had taken up arms. Men and women, lay people and religious, were arriving in ever-growing numbers; others were being taken away and many of them were never seen again. People who were of high rank in Tibetan society were freed. In contrast, three or four young men who attempted to escape were immediately beaten and their bodies were riddled with bullets and left a long time in full view of the other prisoners. They put handcuffs on us and I noticed these were inscribed with tiny letters: 'USA'. We were locked in a large room and once a day they brought us a handful of *tsampa* and some black tea. The soldiers had made off with most of the grain that had been stored in the Tsarong family's cellar.

On 14 March, 1959 (the year pig-earth), they separated me from the others and brought me into an adjacent room. I learned then that hundreds of prisoners had been penned in the gardens of the Tsarong house. At first sight, it appeared there were three or four hundred of us. Some of us, myself included, had succeeded in keeping their *malas*, our prayer beads, and were praying in silence. We all believed that our days were numbered. I remember seeing seriously wounded people, whose wails of pain we could hear at night. Sometimes a piercing cry would travel through the building, followed by an unbearable silence. Someone, perhaps a child, had just died. All around us Tibetans were passing out or screaming suddenly. They would be finished off with a cudgel or an electric truncheon.

I was placed in isolation. Twenty days passed like this and I kept asking myself what they could reproach me for. For being a Tibetan and the Dalai Lama's doctor? It was clear that the Chinese suspected me of something serious. Then one morning a group of us were taken to Chonjuk, while others were directed to the house of the Taring family. Chonjuk? Most of the people of Lhasa had believed that this was a military camp. Perhaps it was, at the beginning of the Chinese occupation. Tibetans had been recruited to help in its construction. In fact they had built their own jail. Chonjuk was an immense rectangular building encircled by barbed wire. Soldiers guarded the entrace, others manned the observation posts. The cells contained between ten and twenty prisoners and were aligned one behind the other. A stream crossed the courtyard. The aristocrats were kept at a distance from the rest of us.

I was pushed into a cell, a vast room where about twenty Tibetans, standing around a central pillar, shot me panicked looks. There were bars on the single window. The floor was covered in wood and the ceiling was decorated with delicate Tibetan motifs.

Toward the middle of the morning a soldier, probably an officer, appeared, accompanied by a Tibetan interpreter. He asked if we had family in Lhasa. Some were allowed to return home under escort to get a blanket and some clothes. Families were also authorized to bring a small package to their relatives. This was at the beginning of our incarceration; later such things became impossible.

When I stated that I lived in Chang-Sep-Char, the tone of the Chinese became more peremptory: 'You, stay there!'

An hour later, they gave cotton blankets to five of my companions and me. The first day at Chonjuk our emotions swung between doubt that this could really be happening and interminable moments of anguish. At eleven o'clock at night the cells were bolted shut and they ordered us to go to sleep. That night, aching with fear, we pressed against each other so we could sleep. At seven o'clock the next day, they woke us and the doors were unbolted. They served us a half-bowl of black tea and a little *tsampa*.

At precisely nine o'clock our door was brutally shoved

open. The same man as the day before appeared, flanked by the translator and another Chinese. They made us sit in a half-circle at the back of the cell.

'We are going to begin the long work of re-education. When you are interrogated, give precise answers. If you lie, you will be punished.'

These first interrogations concerned our lives, our families, our relations. We endured an onslaught of questions to which we were sometimes incapable of responding. For myself, I was only a simple doctor and I knew nothing of the politics of our government. The interrogation of a prisoner would last six to seven hours a day. The victim was made to stand in the middle of the room, next to the pillar. His companions participated in the interrogation and, in fact, we Tibetans were supposed to accuse each other of wrong-doing. This is what the Chinese call *thamzing*.*

Then my turn came. My childhood in the village and in the monastery of Chothey revealed no political involvement on my part but my name had been noticed because I was the Dalai Lama's personal physician and because I lived in the Yapchi family's house, at Chang-Sep-Char. The questions were coming in rapid fire.

'Tenzin Choedrak, what were you doing at Norbulingka? What were you doing in the Yapchis' house? What did the Dalai Lama tell you? You're a spy in the pay of our enemy. What relations did you have with this bandit? What are your other connections?'

I persisted in telling them the only facts that I knew: I was a doctor and my role consisted of caring for patients, and this included the Dalai Lama. The tension grew as the hours went by. Every day we endured an uninterrupted flood of questions. Our jailers designated two or three 'prefects' in each cell. After that it was practically impossible to exchange the least word without it being reported to the guards. The atmosphere among the prisoners became more painful and many succumbed to the pressure. During my second interrogation my companions' behavior toward me changed radically. The translator was urging them to accuse me:

'At the age of fourteen, you were at Chothey and you established relations with such and such persons. Who are they? What did you speak about? What were you thinking? Your responses are not adequate. You are a spy.' Then he would address the others: 'The rest of you, what do you have to say? Tenzin Choedrak is a spy, isn't he?'

Harangued and abused, my cell mates started to accuse me.

'I lied,' avowed a young Tibetan. 'Tenzin Choedrak plotted against the motherland.'

Others pointed threatening fingers at me.

'He's a spy, a spy . . .'

Standing in the middle of the room, I was supposed to detail my life story all over again, but this time adding atrocities. It was horrible. The prisoners around me were becoming agitated. I felt they were ready to save their own skins and that I had become the ideal target.

The interpreter asked me:

'Why didn't you accompany Kundun to India in nineteen fifty-six? What orders did you receive then? On whose behalf were you spying? What were your contacts with the Tibetan resistance? Were you paid by the Kuomintang? Who trained you in espionage? Was it in Calcutta in nineteen fifty-two? What was your relationship with Gyalwa Dondup, the Dalai Lama's brother?'

I always answered the same thing: I was a doctor, I had never spied, and in 1952 I was in Kalimpong caring for *Amala*.

'You're the dog of this renegade the Dalai Lama and his government. If you persist in lying, we will have to chain you up. If you collaborate, we'll let you go.'

There were now two groups of prisoners, the collaborators, who underwent perfunctory interrogations, and the rest of us, who endured the full force of the *thamzing* sessions. Since I occupied the fifth rank in the Tibetan hierarchy, the Chinese said that I had to know what went on in the government and they absolutely insisted that I was in the confidence of high state officials. They said that the Dalai Lama was the cause of all our ills. They accused him of stealing from the people, of sullying the honor of the Tibetans. However, I changed not a word of my account. I could never have denigrated His Holiness the Dalai Lama, our protector and our spiritual guide. I would never have given in! In the evening in the cell I prayed for death to take me soon.

While the officer harangued me with questions, the translator pushed the eighteen others to exhort me to respond. They accused me of receiving money from the Kuomintang, distributing propaganda newspapers, and plotting with the Dalai Lama against the motherland. But I did not hate my fellow Tibetans for it. If they had not participated in this cruel sordid game, they would have been the ones interrogated. And more and more they let themselves be taken in by the game; they invented new stories about me every day. My most serious crime was having been close to the Dalai Lama. The Chinese noted everything, even the smallest detail.

Every morning around seven o'clock they brought us out of the cell. The guards lined up up and led us out of the camp to the nearby river where we could bathe and wash our clothes. How long ago were the days when as adolescents we swam in the Kyitchou and played our games. That was before the invasion, already so long ago . . .

At the beginning of April great news reached me. One of our guards who was positioned a few steps from me was listening to the radio. I heard that Kundun had crossed the border into India on 30 March, and had immediately announced the creation of a government in exile and denounced the 'Seventeen Point Accord'. When I heard this I was filled with joy and I wanted to shout. The prisoner next to me at the riverside was a pleasant-looking person. Plunging my face into a handful of water, I murmured the happy news to him. This thoughtless act was to be my ruin.

Three days later the Chinese organized an important *thamzing* session at which all the prisoners were present. Three heavy machine guns were trained on us. We felt a dull anguish. Perhaps this was the end?

An officer started to speak:

'There are traitors to your cause among you. Subversives have put out the rumor that this renegade the Dalai Lama, this wolf in monk's robes, has set up a government in exile. They've asked that you keep quiet. This is an unacceptable error. You are going to have to pay!'

The prisoners all looked around, each questioned himself and then saw the fault in his immediate neighbor, be it the friend from yesterday, a cousin, a brother. A great clamor started. The officer brought Loguiel, the commander-in-chief of the Tibetan army, out of the ranks. The session of self-criticism could begin. It was going to be terrible for him and for another, Kelsang Ngaouang. The two of them were jeered at and humiliated. It was the Tibetans who struck the blows as the two men stood, in handcuffs, on a platform so they could be seen better. They were soon bleeding and bruised. The Chinese remained unperturbed. Some of the prisoners refused to mistreat their compatriots. But if they did not take part in the onslaught or were seen glancing with compassion at the beaten prisoner, if they allowed themselves a simple fluttering of the eyelid, a slight tic, they in turn endured the *thamzing*. And whoever was beaten like this saw himself automatically isolated by the others.

'Tenzin Choedrak.'

As I came forward I understood that I had been turned in by the man at the river. The superior officer looked at me with hatred, while one of his subordinates led the interrogation.

'You're the one who started this stupid rumor about a government in exile. You're the one who said that "like the slow rotation of the earth, the truth will finally triumph in Tibet." Stupid Tenzin Choedrak!'

I was supposed to keep my eyes on the ground.

'Look at this man!' the officer commanded me.

I raised my head. It was the informer, who was now pointing an accusing finger at me as he told in detail what I had confided to him in the secret joy that I had allowed myself to express. The prisoners accused me again of all the troubles. The informer demanded my immediate execution as a traitor to Tibet.

'He's so obstinate and so reactionary that he deserves to die!' were his words.

That day no-one struck me but they shackled me with chains and a heavy iron bar that caused me horrible pain as soon as I made the slightest movement. When the session came to an end, most of the prisoners were returned to their cells in small groups. Only Loguiel, Kelsang Ngaouang, and I remained on the platform. Some of the Tibetans glared at us as they passed. It pained me so to see them behave like that. Doubtless they knew little about the Dharma! I felt more pity than hatred for them.

They took us to isolation cells, which had small iron doors with peepholes through which they passed our water and meals. My cell was next to the kitchens. Every two or three days, a Chinese and an interpreter would come to ask me:

'Have you reflected? You remember your past actions? Have you finally recovered your memory? Now what do you think? Confess, it'll go better for you.'

Every time I would answer that I had nothing more to say.

'I can't say anything more.'

'You're a zealot, Tenzin Choedrak, but we'll break you. If we have to, we'll execute you, because you have deceived your compatriots.'

One month, perhaps two, had passed since my arrest, I was not quite sure. By then, the Chinese were applying a new policy of repression that consisted of passing off former members of the government and other important persons as thieves. There was an office that dealt with theft and it organized public meetings in Shol, the quarter of Lhasa that was just at the foot of the

Potala. Many Tibetans were publicly humiliated at these sessions in front of their family and their friends. The crowd, confused by what the Chinese were telling them, would fall into the trap. Kelsang Ngaoung was thus taken out of Chonjuk and dragged in chains to the roll of drums to the place where the *thamzing* was to take place. He was accused by the Tibetans who were won over to the cause of the occupiers of having robbed and beaten them. The Chinese encouraged these men and women and congratulated them for their patriotism. The next day Kelsang was brought to Shol. In the meantime, the Chinese had instructed the 'patriots' and told them exactly how they should agitate the crowd against the prisoner. They offered presents, money, carpets, clothing and other valuable objects that had been confiscated from the aristocracy. Kelsang was strongly advised not to respond to the accusations but, better still, to confirm them. Standing motionless, his head lowered, he endured the worst outrages.

'Thief! Bandit!' the crowd shouted.

'Agent of the scoundrel Dalai Lama,' cried a Chinese.

'Kill him! Kill him!' the crowd continued.

Certainly there were Tibetan people who were not duped. Some knew the accused persons, and others were aware of the duplicity of the Chinese. But the Dalai Lama's reputation was damaged and the prisoners, turned over to the fury of the Red Guards, returned to their cells bruised and bleeding. The worst was the shame of still being alive after having denied His Holiness. Some hanged themselves, others tried to escape, with the sole objective of being shot down. And while the Tibetans were going at each other, the Chinese were waiting for the propitious moment to intervene. 'Don't touch him! This is not what the motherland asks of you! Be proud patriots, but do not use violence against dogs.'

I remained in isolation for four weeks. For the last days Loguiel was put in with me. In the evening we recited mantras. During rare moments we could exchange a few words of support, and I especially remember the goodness of this man and his loyalty to his sovereign. We spoke of our compatriots and the torment into which our country had been dragged.

The Chinese published propaganda newspapers that we were forced to read to help in our 're-education'. My mind was very dark. In the silence of the night, troubled by the death-rattles of the wounded, or the shouts of those who were being beaten, I thought about the outrageous demands made by the Popular Army of Liberation. I tried to understand the behavior of our jailers and of some of the prisoners. That discouraged me even more. However, knowing that Kundun was safe and well in India, I hoped in spite of everything that the truth would finally triumph. If not, was it not better that death take me? In the course of one of those nights I promised myself never to insult the memory of the Dalai Lama or his family, even at the peril of my life. Although the Chinese inflicted much suffering on me, I had decided never to give them the pleasure of yielding to them.

I encountered in prison a man who was from Hor, which is in the north-east of Tibet. This man refused to give in to the guards' demands that we revile the Dalai Lama's name. He came from a very poor region and, unlike me, had never met His Holiness. The Chinese considered his attitude completely crazy, if not suicidal.

But he told me that he could not act badly toward our sovereign, who had never betrayed him. If he must die, he said, it would be with a pure spirit. I did not see him again after this encounter. Doubtless he was executed. But his attitude came from a simple respect of the universal morality. The people of Hor used to sing this as they went about their work:

> *Acceptance is like wearing*
> *A hat of wet leather.*
> *The more time passes,*
> *The more the hat fits the head.*

My cell neighbor's name was Tsarong. He could not bear the moral and physical tortures that he was put through and he committed suicide. How could one blame him for it? He was not the only one at Chonjuk to make an attempt on his life, even though as Buddhists we are opposed to such extremes. Thousands of ill-omened thoughts crossed my mind, but in spite of everything, I succeeded in appeasing them through prayers. Also, I had managed to keep my *mala*, which was my most precious possession. My only possessions were in fact these prayer beads and the knowledge of medicine that Khenrab Norbu had imparted to me. Other Tibetans owned land, money, sometimes much gold. In order to take my possessions from me, they would have to kill me; the rich were only robbed. I remember that the rich families of Lhasa and its surroundings had brought many of their possessions to the Potala and to the monastery of Drepoung, which were considered safe places when the country was threatened. As soon as the Dalai Lama left, the Chinese

174

invaded the palace and razed the monasteries, seizing especially the sacred works, but also all the gold and all the silver of the nobility. They carried them off to China by the roads that we had been forced to build. In prison, I met several Tibetans who had been robbed of their most precious objects and their lands, which were redistributed to the people in the name of the Communist doctrine. Here are two examples. One family had hidden all its gold in an old worn box, and, to deceive thieves, had filled shiny new boxes with pebbles, assuming those would be the ones to be taken. In the course of a house search, soldiers found at least forty kilos of precious metals that they carried off laughing all the way, as the head of the family was led away to Chonjuk. Another family had the same experience. By using metal detectors, the soldiers this time found the gold hidden under the floor. This shows how naive the Tibetans were, also to what extent they let themselves be hoodwinked by the Communists' inflamed speeches. Did our people still have a debt to pay? But what debt did they owe to the Chinese?

At night, Loguiel and I would practice *kyapdro*: taking refuge in the three Joys that are the Buddha, the Dharma, and the Sangha.* We devoted ourselves to it with so much ardor that soon we had surpassed a hundred thousand recitations.

After four weeks of isolation, they separated me from Loguiel. One morning a Chinese officer opened the door and said:

'Tenzin Choedrak, have you reflected?'

'I have nothing to add to what I've told you,' I answered him wearily.

At a simple nod of his head six guards took hold of

me and dragged me out. They led me into the common cell where I found my former companions. There were twenty-three of them, seated at the back of the room on cotton mattresses, obviously waiting for me. The officer stood to one side, the translator next to him, as well as a secretary who would write down everything I was going to say. Then began a very painful session of *thamzing*. I was standing in the middle of the room.

'Confess! Do you realize what you're doing? Confess!' they were shouting.

'I have reflected carefully. I have nothing to add to my statements. I am not a spy, I have never worked for the Kuomintang. I have told you the truth. I have always tried to follow the Dharma. You accuse me of being in the pay of the Dalai Lama? What fault has he committed for you to act this way? In what act of espionage have I taken part?'

The Tibetans all stood up and looked very threatening.

'You are a reactionary and stubborn. It is we, by the grace of the Han, who belong to the great motherland. You're the type who prefers to throw himself off a cliff.'

The officer advised me again to confess, but I said I had already told the truth and had nothing else to add. At a sign from him, the guards tied me to a wooden board with a heavy rope. When they tightened it, the board pressed into my back and broke the skin. I was bleeding and in terrible pain. It was my own countrymen, including some I had cared for, who struck the first blows. Is that not unbelievable? The Chinese stayed out of it and watched the scene with amusement. I was punched and kicked with the point of their thin rubber shoes which added to the pain. I was bleeding profusely. They hit me in the head, the stomach, on the legs, aiming for the most sensitive parts of the body. My mouth bled and I felt my teeth coming loose. I cannot say how long the beating went on, but before falling unconscious I prayed to be purified of all my bad kharmic imprints. It was then that one of them wrote a letter with my own blood demanding my execution. Among the twenty-three prisoners, I remember Tenzin Gyaltsen and Tsenam, who were forced to hit me, but I knew perfectly well they were holding back. They are among the few witnesses who are still able to tell what happened at Chonjuk in that period. Today they work by my side at Men-Tsee-Khang in Dharamsala.

Then came the black hole. They carried me on a stretcher to an isolation cell. Loguiel was gone. I remained in a semi-coma for several days. When I came to I was unable to open my eyes or speak and I had great difficulty breathing. My entire body was covered in wounds and contusions, my mouth clotted with blood on which flies settled. The guards were convinced for a long time that I was going to die. I thought so too, and in some ways I hoped I would. They called a doctor who examined me and told them that I did not have long and that there was nothing he could do for me. I was thirsty, my throat burned. My body and my clothes reeked. No-one took care of me for fear of bringing the same punishment down on themselves. The officers had given the order to the guards that if I died, the prisoners should be blamed, and not to say I was tortured.

My conscience dictated to me that in spite of all I should resist and struggle as much as possible. I prayed day and night and I repeated endlessly the *kyapdro*. In order to keep track of the number of prayers I had recited, I pulled out threads from the mattress and made one knot for every prayer.

A little more than four months had gone by. The summer of 1959 was coming to an end. I survived and remained in complete isolation until the end of my incarceration at Chonjuk.

12

In the Hell of the Chinese Prisons

My stay at Chonjuk ended in October 1959. It was getting colder and so the conditions of our detention became harsher. I was chained night and day in my cell. My mattress was worn and caked with my blood. In some places, the cotton had bunched together and had hardened in uneven balls which gave me much discomfort when I tried to sleep. It was the same when I sat. At night I tried to warm my feet by rubbing them against each other, which was not easy to do because of the iron bar that bound my ankles.

Throughout my isolation I had tried in vain to understand the behavior of those of my compatriots who were ready to do anything to satisfy the least demand of our occupiers. They doubtless hoped to be rewarded by the Communist system. As for the Chinese, even if I am a Buddhist monk committed to non-violence, I can understand that soldiers perpetrate all sorts of atrocities in obeying orders. In contrast, I feel infinite sadness about the Tibetans who beat their own to death to win favors from our occupiers. Even if the Chinese manipulated and put pressure on them, some of them showed far more zeal than needed. There was still another category of Tibetans: those who touted pro-Chinese sentiments with the goal of escaping torture. For them I feel no anger, and I prefer to pray for them so that they may return to the path of the Dharma.

Psychologically I sometimes felt discouraged to the point of losing all hope. His Holiness was gone and Tibet had been transformed into a vast field of horror where bloodbaths ran. I felt that my country was like an orphaned child crying for its absent mother. It was pitiful. The only news we received in prison were glowing reports about China by Mao, which presented Tibetan society as backward and feudal. Certainly it had its faults and it was backward in many ways, but our government had been paying attention to our desire for modernization and profound change. Kundun had begun to undertake reforms before the invasion in 1949; we had no need for China. However sad the situation was, I tried to believe that the evil would come to an end. But the months passed and Kundun was unable to return.

One morning, I was led into a tent full of officers who were protected by armed soldiers. They put me in the center. A Chinese, visibly the highest ranking, said to me:

'Tenzin Choedrak, you must talk. Tell us what you know about your government's policies.'

'I have already answered all your questions. I'm a doctor, and I have nothing to add,' I insisted.

'Times have changed,' the man continued. 'You must give your allegiance to the motherland. Tibet is today a thing of the past. From now on the future belongs to you, with us, for the good of the Tibetan people.'

'I can't change my position, since I've already told you

the truth,' I answered. 'If I said the opposite, I'd be lying. Anyway, I'm Tibetan, not Chinese . . .'

'Tenzin Choedrak, you still can't tell the difference between good and evil.'

I told them that we did not have the same perception of good and evil. They sent me back to isolation but this time I was not beaten. A few days later they gathered the prisoners in the large room where the *thamzing* sessions took place. The soldiers divided us into three groups: the first were all who accepted life under Chinese guardianship; the second, all who pretended indifference or who approved in silence the Chinese presence; and finally, the group in which they placed me, those who were faithful to the Tibetan cause and to His Holiness the Dalai Lama. A funtionary spoke to us:

'Some of you are going to leave soon for China to be re-educated. Hard work is waiting for you there because you have immature brains. You,' and he pointed at the first two groups, 'you will work on the construction of an electrical power station. As for you,' and he looked scornfully at us, 'you will be leaving to finish your re-education.'

On 28 October I left Chonjuk and was transferred with seventy-two other prisoners to the military prison of Jiuzhen. We had no baggage, only the rags that we were wearing. Relatives were authorized to come and speak to us for a few minutes. I could converse a little with members of my family. All around we heard weeping and moaning. It was emotional and painful. As soon as the meetings ended we saw a group of the prisoners whom the Chinese used for their dirty work. If we were obstinate in our behavior they insulted us and threatened us with death. This time they spat on us and whipped us under the indifferent gaze of the guards.

We were not far from the Potala. From the window of our cell we could even glimpse it. Would we see it again one day? We huddled together and spent a large part of the night praying. During the night a violent storm broke over the capital and the rain whipped the ground with extreme violence. When lightning tore the sky, the Dalai Lama's palace appeared, like a vision of hope. We were convinced that in one, two, three, even five years at most, Kundun would be back in Lhasa and that a long period of peace with our Chinese neighbors would follow.

Day had scarcely broken when they herded us into two trucks. Four armed soldiers guarded us and an officer took up a position next to each driver. A third truck containing the soldiers' provisions and tents was going to precede us into China. Soldiers were also posted in this truck from which a heavy machine gun remained permanently aimed at us. Two Tibetans acted as interpreters.

Orders were given and the trucks started up. The last image I had of Lhasa was the Potala, adorned with a magnificent double rainbow that rose in the west of the mountains and dispersed in the dark clouds in the east. Another storm was threatening.

The trip to the prison of Jiuzhen took twelve days. Standing pressed against each other and chained from head to foot, there was no possibility of moving. Falling down would have meant death.

The convoy set out in the direction of Nagtchou. As we left Lhasa we were joined by another vehicle carrying monks from Drepoung, Ganden and Sera.

They could not have been more than sixteen years old. Around noon, they gave us a handful of rice and some black tea. At the end of the afternoon, the officers ordered the vehicles to stop. We were at Amdo Teuma, which was entirely desert land. They had the tents erected and put us in one of them. It was horribly cold, a violent wind was battering the mountain and it began to snow heavily. Although we huddled together, we still could not get warm. Some began to weep. Their moans immediately unleashed the guards' anger. Out of fear the young monks urinated on themselves.

I could not sleep in such conditions. My mind wandered from thoughts about my country, which I was about to leave, to feelings of compassion for the young Chinese soldiers who stood guard outside in the storm. I would have liked to say a few words to them about their country, about my country, to speak to them about Kundun, who was the same age as them.

I remember also a man among us who was from the Amdo. He was ill and lost consciousness several times. The Chinese paid hardly any attention to him and he was subjected to the same regime as the rest of us. One life more or less mattered little to them. We spent two nights in the tent. The third day we crossed a mountain pass by which we reached To To Ga. It was there that the guards threw the sick man out of the truck and left him for dead. He was young and I was convinced that he was still alive. I implored Tara to protect him. Sometimes we encountered nomads but we were forbidden to look at them. If we were caught we received a mean blow in the back with a rifle butt.

Then we traveled across the plain of Gharmu where we crossed a caravan of goats returning from the high salt lakes. Very far away on the horizon we could make out Tibetan prisoners who were breaking up stones. I learned later that China was extracting oil from the region. After Gharmu, we reached Tsadam; there was salt everywhere, on the sides of the road, and around the houses, and no potable water anywhere. The salt, cold and snow were bad enough, but at the end of this trip, which lasted another three days, a real hell was waiting for us.

We were now in China. We made the last leg of the trip by train locked in a boxcar. The Chinese had separated us from the monks from Drepoung who left for another destination, another camp. We were all in a state of extreme weakness. There was among us a young lama from Pangbo who was incredibly naive. The Chinese had let him belive that he was going to China to study. He was seated next to me in the train, and he assured me that he would not return to Tibet until he had finished his studies. I did not dare inform him of the probable fate that was waiting for us at the end of this train line. Later at Jiuzhen a few of the prisoners teased him:

'So! You're staying with us a little while for your studies?'

He would turn away his head to hide his embarrassment.

A very long night had just passed. The train was heading for Beijing, which was a day's distance, but for us the trip ended in the outskirts of Jiuzhen. The boxcar doors were pulled open and we were ordered out. From there trucks took us to the camp.

Jiuzhen was situated in the middle of vast fields and was surrounded by barbed wire. Three other prisons in the area belonged to this camp. The main entrance was on the east side. On either side of the entrance there was a row of five cells; two other rows of ten cells each, parallel to the entrance, were separated by a large courtyard. In the back were the kitchens, and here and there, wooden huts for the cesspits. Soldiers were posted in different parts of the camp. They occupied a building situated outside the enclosure. Escape was said to be impossible but there had been a few attempts via the cesspits which opened onto the back of the camp. Since then the guards were more vigilant.

The cell doors were made of heavy wood; the beds were fashioned of wood and grass, which we tried to cover with pieces of cloth. The cells were built to hold five prisoners but there could be as many as seven. There were other cells that held as many as twenty-five prisoners. The overcrowding frequently provoked horrible fights. Everybody marked his territory by drawing lines on the floor and woe to him who crossed them.

At Jiuzhen there were some eight hundred prisoners, among them Chinese political prisoners, formerly of the Kuomintang, and anti-Communists. Other Chinese, Catholics and Muslims were imprisoned here for not respecting the ban on religious practice. There were also seven women who occupied a cell a little off to the side. Three hundred Tibetans, most of them from the Amdo region, had already been transferred to this camp. By the time we arrived there were only two survivors; all the others had died of starvation or from torture. One of the two, Aki Lama, was a young *tulku* who could stand only with difficulty. When I saw him for the first time he must have been barely eighteen years old. His companion in misfortune was a layman from the Amdo who was about thirty years old. Both were in a pitiful state.

The new arrivals were gathered in the courtyard, and the head of the camp ordered the rules to be read. Most of the guards were Chinese but there were also some Tibetans, former prisoners who had 'converted' or had collaborated from the start, who showed fierce resentment toward us. The seventy-two prisoners were divided into three groups and directed to the cells in the main building.

The first day at Jiuzhen they got us up at seven o'clock. An hour later a Tibetan explained to us the work we were supposed to do. The guards shouted their orders from the loudspeakers which could be heard from the furthest point of the camp. I noticed then that the prisoners who collaborated occupied a special barracks close to that of their masters.

With empty stomachs we were led to a distant field. There we were supposed to fill sacks with sand and carry them to another spot. Whoever failed to meet the quota of thirty sacks a day was automatically denied the next meal. From the first day some of my companions who were further weakened by the journey from Lhasa to Jiuzhen received no nourishment. At noon we were given their portion of rice. We could then rest for an hour during which we were allowed to sleep, a favor we quickly appreciated. Afterwards we went back to the field until dinner, which was served at six o'clock.

Winter was fearsome in Jiuzhen. A whirling wind swept the plain and made the work in the fields even more difficult. They passed out hats and gloves to us which we stuffed with cotton. In the evening in the cell we wrapped our feet with dirty rags, also stuffed with cotton. Food was almost non-existent. Our monthly ration consisted of four kilos of rice and dried vegetables, which scarcely sustained us and obviously could not satisfy even the most minimal needs. Malnutrition quickly got the better of the hardiest of us. Personally I was not in excellent health when I arrived at Jiuzhen and after a few days of hard labor I lost even more weight and rapidly became terribly thin. But I was not the worst off. Because of our weakness we walked very slowly; it could take several seconds to raise a leg, several more to take a step. Some of us had to hold onto the wall to stand up. No-one was allowed to help the weakest and they received no care. There was a building referred to as the 'hospital', but it was only a ruse. Life in Jiuzhen was miserable. Our bodies were swollen like inflated tubes and our hair fell out in clumps.

In the evenings we underwent a special 're-education' session. First the jailers accused us, then mistreated us for our past conduct. The most resistant prisoners were shamed for not being patriots:

'You are reactionaries and we will break you. Either you admit your faults or you die.'

They beat us until we bled. Whoever persisted in resisting was sent into isolation, a dreadful fate. There we were deprived of food and endured the worst outrages. On Sundays they taught us the principles of Marxism with Chinese Communist commentary. An officer read to us from Mao's Little Red Book as though this were a sacred text. The methods at Jiuzhen were like those at Chonjuk, and all the other prisons in China and Tibet. But unlike Chonjuk, here they beat and tortured us and also set the prisoners against each other. They were so proficient that they could end the torture just before the victim's heart would have stopped. They much preferred to finish him off by forced labor.

After a few weeks of detention at Jiuzhen we all suffered from malnutrition. Many prisoners ate whatever they could find, leather, cotton, pieces of their clothes. Some of the Chinese prisoners went so far as looking for worms in the latrines. A servant of the Yapchi family, who was in the camp with me at that time, found a jacket on the ground which he cooked and devoured. Such behavior became more and more common.

Regularly on our return from the field, we were beaten. Our Tibetan jailers, with the others, reproached us for not putting enough ardor into our work for the motherland. And their Chinese accomplices accused us of barbarous acts, which they themselves were actually committing: 'You oppressed the worker masses, you drank their blood and ate their flesh.'

There have never been any cases of cannibalism among Tibetans, which is far from the case in China. Whatever our condition, the guards took no notice. On the contrary, the weaker we were, the more they abused us. Our lives were consumed by work in the fields, torture, and re-education.

A monk from the northern part of Tibet, surprised by soldiers in the prayer room of his monastery while he was praying, had been arrested a long time ago. The Chinese had proposed to him that he go to work in China, which he readily accepted. A few days later this man found himself in Jiuzhen. Now he was full of regret. The Chinese used him like a beast of burden, forcing him to do the very painful tasks. Tortured several times a week, the poor monk quickly weakened and succumbed to the mistreatment.

I was now part of another group of prisoners whose task was to clear and then cultivate an acre of scrub terrain. The ground was frozen and we had to dig deep into the earth to be able to plant the seeds. The skin of our hands was raw, our feet blistered and swollen. The oldest ones among us who could not endure this regime contracted illnesses and died. The health of Aki Lama also deteriorated. He called us all *akhou*, which means 'uncle', and a little smile would appear on his lips when we were able to help him discreetly back to his cell. A Tibetan who collaborated with the Chinese even took pity on him. Every day he tried to give him back a little strength by spooning some vegetable stock mixed with flour into his mouth. But it was already too late. Death soon took Aki Lama.

I found plants in the fields that possessed medicinal properties and distributed them to my companions. A guard noticed, however, and threatened me with *thamzing*.

A new year began. It was 1960 (the year mouse-iron), and the Chinese knew that we would have liked to celebrate *Lossar*, the Tibetan new year. Some officers came into the cell at dinner time and said:

'You have drunk the blood and the sweat of the Tibetan people. Nevertheless, the Communists are happy to offer this oil to you today as a gift to celebrate the new year. We hope you will change your attitude toward the mother country and will acknowlege your errors.'

Famished, some prisoners asked for a little more oil.

'You were too privileged when you had your freedom. You don't deserve it, but for this once . . .'

The man poured a little more oil into each of the bowls but the vegetables we had been served to augment the handful of rice were rotten.

The next day one of our companions, Lobsang Dhondrup, was supposed to go with a team to pick up some manure and spread it in the fields. I ws also part of this detail. Suddenly, he signaled to me.

'Look! Dead piglets,' he whispered to me.

'Don't touch them,' I said to him. 'You're going to get in trouble.'

He did not listen to me and continued to gather the manure. The carcasses gave off a strong odor of decay and one of them had a gash on the body. He slipped one of them out of the hole where they lay and concealed it.

I tried to reason with him: 'Don't do that. You're going to get sick and bring trouble on yourself.'

'I absolutely must eat. Whatever happens, I have to eat. I can't stand this any more.'

As he was about to take the animal into his cell he was caught. The guards confiscated the carcass and he was beaten all night. His shouts echoed around the camp and got into our bones. In the early morning they transported him to the hospital where he died from the torture.

I could give many more examples of the malnutrition that was everywhere in Jiuzhen. One day another of my companions, Niepama Tenzin, noticed that the Chinese had thrown some soup on the ground. It had run down to the sewer outlet where all sorts of debris floated in it. Everybody who entered the kitchen had walked in it. Despite all my warnings, Niepama Tenzin rushed to the spot and filled his bowl with this horrible mixture.

'This soup is made from mule-meat stock,' he said excitedly.

Others ate rats that they cooked on a stripped electric wire. This was nothing compared to what awaited us. At the time, famine was so terrible in China that adolescents were driven to appalling extremes. One of the camp prisoners had killed his mother to steal four kilos of rice from her and had been sentenced to seventeen years in the camp. Another had killed and eaten a newborn. We called him 'the vulture' because in Tibet we give cadavers to the birds of prey.

Spring finally brought more clement days. My spirits were lifted but I was also extremely weak. To lie down I did like the others. I first placed my head on the mattress, then I gradually stretched out. Some could not even lift their heads. All my joints ached and intense pain pierced my back. Getting up was another matter and it took me for ever. I would grip the wall and little by little unfold my bruised body. We no longer even had the energy to control our defecations and we urinated on ourselves. In the beginning I could still manage to use my bowl but later I could no longer control myself.

In Jiuzhen I often thought about dying. It was what happened to most of my companions. My two neighboring companions in the cell were called Kire Cheupel and Dodroung Tsewang Rapguiel. It was two o'clock in the morning one day when I noticed that Cheupel had died. Dodroung and I immediately decided to conceal his death from the guards in order to get his soup portion which we shared greedily. That same morning the cook, a strong and vigorous Tibetan, had hidden a little soup in an empty cell. I noticed it and stole it to share with my friends. When the cook came back he was furious. It was not very serious for him because, unlike us, he could eat to satisfy his hunger. Cheupel's body remained in the cell a part of the morning, then we carried him to the place near the latrines where the dead were piled up. There were several deaths every day and the prisoners were supposed to take turns burying the dead. The bodies sometimes stayed near the latrines for a few days before being brought outside the camp to a field specially set aside for this purpose. The Chinese had the name of the dead person inscribed on the spot where he was buried.

In spite of everything I survived, doubtless a little better than the others because I knew how to utilize the various resources that nature offered. When I found any nourishing or medicinal plants, I would eat them, and whenever possible I would make a treacle with them that I shared. One of my companions, Trinele Namguiel, was saved from a certain death by swallowing this mixture. We also ate a sort of radish, called *tang*.

We continued to endure long 're-education' sessions in the evenings that always included the reading of Mao Zedong's Little Red Book. The Chinese officers regularly talked about different forms of government. Their principal targets were the Americans, the British, the Indians, and the French, all of whom were labeled imperialists. If we contested their arguments we were traitors and they accused us of wanting to spread anti-Communist propaganda in the camp. The new prisoners frequently fell into the trap. The rest of us listened with approval to everything they cared to tell us.

We also underwent a daily round of *thamzing* in the course of which we were supposed to criticize ourselves. Those who refused to humiliate themselves before the others were accused of trying to hide their faults and were placed in isolation where they were tortured throughout the night. We told lies of all sorts to our tormentors to make them believe the 're-education' had been a success.

In 1961 (the year ox-iron) a Chinese woman came frequently to the prison hospital to exchange cigarettes and a little food for different objects. One day I decided to give up my *chupa* for twenty pieces of *momos**, which are small meat pastries, and a steamed roll stuffed with meat and vegetables. The exchange allowed me one day's respite from the pangs of hunger. The woman was eventually surprised during her bartering by the guards, who punished her, though not too severely. The news of her arrest distressed us and eroded our morale even more.

Another time we noticed the cook carrying a big portion of *momos*. We threw ourselves on him and grabbed it from his hands. Late in the afternoon the guards gathered us in the courtyard. Those of us who had tasted the *momos* were bound; when they pulled on the rope the pain was so intense that we howled and urinated on ourselves. The Chinese appointed the most zealous Tibetan prisoners to carry out this special punishment.

The Chinese prisoners endured the same treatment as the rest of us. Two former directors of the Kuomintang happened to find an ass's head in the camp. Because the brain was intact they ate it. When the guards found out they called a session in the courtyard. The two men had to criticize each other and were physically tortured by the others under the indifferent gaze of the camp officials. Among other horrors, we discovered that a Chinese prisoner had fallen into the cesspit. Had he been pushed by a guard? No-one could say. The smell he gave off was unbearable. A white foam came from his mouth. A soldier arrived and kicked him in the stomach, made him get up and led him into the field where he normally would have been working. That was where he died.

As I have said, having medical knowledge favored me greatly in Jiuzhen. My companions were dying one after the other. Of the seventy-two Tibetans who arrived with me, there were soon not more than fifty, then forty, then thirty. During the first weeks of my incarceration I prayed for the starvation and the suffering to end. I managed to endure the blows, the torture, and the hunger. To help me remain lucid in the moments of extreme pain and physical weakness, I would call to mind teachings such as this one:

> *Do not perpetrate negative actions,*
> *Make the effort to practice virtue,*
> *Apply yourself to master your mind completely,*
> *Such is the teaching of the Buddha.*

The teaching I most often recited was called the *Jampel-Yang Cherap Teunpa*. At Chonjuk I used to say the prayers known as the *kyadpro* and the *Netchoung Soung*. At Jiuzhen I often opened Mao's Little Red Book in the guards' presence but I was actually saying prayers, my own prayers. To be able to survive all that I had to endure in the death camp I also used meditation, notably a particular form called *tougou-bartsa*, which allows one to go without food for a number of days without too much difficulty and without any secondary effect. It produces a specific warmth and this sensation appeases hunger. I do not have the ability to transmit this teaching, which can be received only from a great lama. It was Kham Rinpoche, who is now deceased, who transmitted it to me on his arrival at Loka. This meditation is practiced especially in retreats and is much used by the Tibetan hermits in certain secluded places of Ladakh. I can, however, describe my personal experience of the practice at Jiuzhen. When there was no more light in the cell, I would move away from the other prisoners. For this practice, one does not pray, but simply remains seated in silence. Around me my companions were talking or calling on the divinities, others moaning in pain. I would try to remain calm and quiet, turned completely to my meditation. This practice creates heat in the stomach which is then diffused throughout the body. It helps to carry nutritive elements so it is preferable to eat something before practicing it. This heat also helps the digestion. With an empty stomach the effects are weaker.

According to the ideal of the bodhisattva it is good to come to the aid of our enemy as well as our friend and even to consider our enemy as our dearest relation. Applying that principle is very difficult, especially in the conditions in which we were living. In spite of everything, at Jiuzhen as at Chonjuk, I always tried to respect the words of the Buddha even though I felt resentment toward the Chinese and the Tibetans who tortured us. But I succeeded in distancing this feeling of anger through meditation, prayers, and respect for the teachings of the Dharma.

To encourage us to practice Buddhism, a few profoundly spiritual beings made us confront our misfortunes without bad intentions toward those who inflict these sufferings on us. The great master Aticha says in 'The Light of the Way':

> *He who, on the basis of an understanding of his own*
> * suffering,*
> *Develops the desire to assuage another*
> *For all sorts of suffering*
> *Is qualified as a superior being.*

There are certainly Tibetans, Chinese, and other people who have lived in conditions much more deplorable than ours. In the most difficult moments some great lamas would evoke for us the exemplary lives of Tibetan spiritual masters, who could serve as an example to us and thus help us endure our own suffering. Among these masters one of the most frequently quoted was the great yogi and poet Milarepa, who lived a life of the most complete self-denial, sustaining himself only on thistles gathered in the mountains. Against such austerity we had to agree that we were in a better situation, even if we had to tolerate the *thamzing* sessions and our jailers' brutalities. In the camps I encountered *tulkus* who were capable of tolerance, although they were beaten to the point of death. They shone with a strange serenity. As for me, anger filled me as soon as the blows began to rain down. I did finally succeed in mastering my reaction and even in erasing the very idea of anger from my mind. However, I still had much work to do to acquire the serenity of the *tulkus* in the face of all ordeals. I could see at Jiuzhen Catholic women and Muslims facing suffering with as much tolerance as certain lamas.

I applied the teachings of the Dharma every day and in all circumstances, for I have always had an unshakable faith in Buddhism. It still happened that some well-known lamas in the camps proved to be less than scrupulous. The spiritual practice had become for them a joke. Hunger pushed them to massacre animals. Although they owed respect to all living beings, they deliberately killed pigs, rats, dogs, and cruelly cut up living monkeys to the laughter of the Chinese. Worse still, some served the executioner and beat to death their compatriots who had shown them only respect.

I have observed that suffering produced a curious effect in the lives of some of the prisoners. Those who survived developed a strange and particularly unstable social behavior. Many former prisoners of these Chinese camps ended up as living dead, on the margins of society. They were forever haunted by the years of imprisonment and torture and often gave off a frightening aura. If there were not more cases of madness among us, I believe it was because of the support of religion, our attachment to the Dharma. Considering the desperate conditions in which we existed, instances of suicide were surprisingly rare. For us as Buddhists, it is a privilege to be born human, linked to the actions of our previous lives. To deliberately take leave of this life is an act that may cause great suffering in the lives to come. I cannot blame those who cracked in the Chinese camps. Their sufferings were unimaginable. Some begged their jailers for death, writing their pleas with their own blood on the cell walls.

It is true that I felt anger toward the Communist Chinese, but even more toward the Tibetans, religious and lay, who collaborated with the occupiers. But when one is in a state of anger, contact with reality is lost. Anger has destructive effects, engenders negative thoughts like the desire to inflict more suffering in return. It is by tenacity and patience that one succeeds in dominating these negative forces. When the Chinese or Tibetans tortured me I would lose all ability to reason because anger dominated me. I would slowly calm down and finally succeed in controlling my thoughts and then the physical pain. Meditation, secret exercises that we call *toumo*, and the recitation of mantras permitted me to endure the blows and the electric shocks.

Before describing our departure from China, I am reminded of a Chinese prisoner. We are all human and it is important, not to say essential, to be concerned about each other. The man was suffering from a serious illness. His gangrenous thighs were pullulating with white worms. He moaned continuously. Several times a day, a Chinese Christian nurse came to look after him, covering the wounds on his anus and thighs with ash. This treatment seemed to quiet his pain, but he died very soon. 'The cyclical existence is the cradle in which miseries are born and grow,' said the Great Fifth Dalai Lama.

At the end of 1961 our situation improved. One day they gathered us in the courtyard. Of the seventy-two

Tibetan prisoners who had arrived with me in October 1959, we were now no more than twenty-one.

'Your re-education is at an end,' an officer told us. 'In a few weeks you will return to Tibet.'

That day we could better endure the glacial 'Mongol wind' that could blow for a good twenty minutes at a time. When it let loose, the guards made an announcement through the loudspeakers. You then had to protect yourself and we would run and seek refuge in the shelters dug for this purpose. Two weeks later, the prisoners were called together again. They announced that our rations would be increased from four to twenty kilos a month. We had to be fattened up to withstand the return journey. There was not one among us who was capable of withstanding twelve days in an open truck. No more work in the fields, the weakest could even stay in bed; the others stayed in the cells or sat about outside. We were still subjected to *thamzing* sessions, but gradually our bodies took on a little weight. We could raise our heads a bit more easily, although lying down and standing up were still difficult.

One morning they lined all of us up in the courtyard and the officer announced our departure. A week later, the escort arrived under the command of a Chinese officer and two Tibetan assistants. For the journey they gave us each some toasted wheat flour that they ladled out of a pot. As we had no container to keep it in, we tore up pieces of our pants and fabricated little sacks, tying a knot at one end. Some of the flour had not been cooked sufficiently, but of course we ate it anyway. They told us not to bring anything with us because the Chinese would provide us with everything we needed at Drapchi. This time we did not believe them and we brought along what little we possessed.

Some of the prisoners went to the prison hospital during this last week at Jiuzhen. The doctor gave them oxygen masks and allowed them a few days of rest. Among us there was Jigme Tenzin. He was tubercular and had much difficulty moving. In the course of the first day of the trip he confided in me his anguish and his doubts. Before coming to Jiuzhen Jigme Tenzin had a vision of the sacred lake Lhamo-Latso where the conditions of the rebirth of the thirteenth Dalai Lama had been foreseen. In his vision he saw himself in prison, and then he saw the upper floors of the Potala and his family. I told him this was a good omen and that he would soon see his people again. He maintained that his end was near and he expressed concern about his family. I tried to comfort him and promised to take care of them if anything happened to him. As strange as it seems, his visions were realized. While we were being led to the Drapchi prison, which is in Lhasa, he did in fact see the Potala. Unfortunately, his health deteriorated and he had to be taken to the hospital where he did actually meet his family a last time before dying. Because I was the Dalai Lama's physician, the others were convinced that I would live a long time and many of them confided their last wishes in me before taking leave of their bodies. It was a heavy task that I did not succeed in carrying out until many years later. Out of the seventy-two Tibetans who had left with me for the Jiuzhen camp, today there are now only three survivors.

Shortly before our departure from Jiuzhen the Tibetans were singing this song:

In the Hell of the Chinese Prisons

Akhou, Akhou!
We have known hell.
Free us now,
Free us!

The song was taken up later in Lhasa and the Chinese reaction was terrible.

13

Drapchi: the Death Camp

We arrived in Nagtchou in late afternoon and spent the night in the prison that had been built to house the Tibetan prisoners who were working on road construction. We were roughly crowded into a cell that had been hastily emptied. The room was very dark. It seemed that someone had recently made a fire in there and the floor was littered with goat droppings and shreds of cloth. We rubbed the cotton against the stone floor and by dint of much patience, we finally got some smoke and then a flame that we fed with the goat droppings.

We had been in the cell only a few minutes when Lekdoup, usually very reserved, started to behave strangely: he cautiously scraped the wall with his fingernails, then he sat down, opened up his sack of *tsampa*, mixed it with his precious harvest and ate the whole thing greedily.

'It smells of yak,' another prisoner suddenly remarked.

At that moment we realized that there was *dri* butter stuck to the wall. Our predecessors had probably spread it there to hide it from the guards. That evening, all our sense were alert. We were rediscovering odors that we had not smelled since 1959 when we left Lhasa, but which had been so familiar before. In the neighboring cells some of the prisoners were even cooking meat and drinking Tibetan tea.

At daybreak the next day we headed in the direction of Lhasa and reached the city around ten o'clock at night, on 18 October, 1962 (the year tiger-water). The guards led us to Drapchi, the number one prison, where we were assigned to several cells. The first sound that I heard in this 'death camp' was the inhuman cry of someone being tortured. I closed my eyes and a shudder ran through my body. In the morning the smell of tea with milk filled the prison. The new arrivals received black tea, while the other prisoners drank Tibetan tea, that is, with milk. The black tea caused me horrible stomach pains and uncontrollable diarrhea.

The Chinese authorities soon announced they had not yet made a decision about me. I was still accused of spying but had not been sentenced. My family was told of my arrival at Drapchi. An uncle was able to come and see me for ten minutes. He gave me news of my father and *Mola* and offered me a little butter and some dried yak meat. Although I was reduced to a skeletal state, I tried to sit up straight to reassure my family. In these brief exchanges no-one was deceived, however, since those on the outside were also enduring severe deprivation.

At Drapchi the wake-up call was at seven o'clcok. One morning, they gathered the twenty-one prisoners from Jiuzhen in a large room. An officer told us to prepare to give an accounting of our three years in China.

'Some among you persist in not recognizing the values of Communism. You must do so or you will die here.'

There was no *thamzing* session but that changed the next day. I was still considered strong-minded so a special regime was reserved for me. I was chained and made to kneel on sharp stones; facing the other prisoners, I was ordered to recount my faults and ask for forgiveness, while the guards, seated on wooden chairs, enjoyed my humiliation. My knees became running sores. Throughout I refused to condemn the Dalai Lama and his family.

The victim of a *thamzing* session that had gotten out of control could not be left to die in the prison but would be taken to the hospital in Lhasa. The authorities wanted everyone to believe that the Tibetans were very bellicose among themselves and that the guards would have to intervene regularly to separate them. Once a week all the prisoners were assembled in the courtyard for an accusation session during which the Chinese read the names of those who had confessed their 'crimes'.

One of the most repugnant tasks that they assigned to the recalcitrant consisted of killing flies in the cesspits. Armed with a fine bamboo stick on the end of which was fastened a piece of thick paper, they hit the flies as soon as they landed on the excrement. Some prisoners claimed they killed more than a thousand a day.

Every week they made us read propaganda newspapers that touted the virtues of the economic system of the motherland. We would read that the Tibetans were now living happily and willingly worked their land at night by the light of lamps. They also said food production surpassed the total volume of the Matchouo (Huangho) and Dritchou (Yangtse) rivers. All that was, of course, nothing but lies. In reality, the Chinese requisitioned the grain for the troops, and the Tibetan people were dying of hunger.

At Drapchi I opted for a different attitude than at Jiuzhen: I kept quiet and behaved in ways that enabled me to avoid the guards' wrath. I was beaten less than at Chonjuk or Jiuzhen. Since food was provided more consistently than in the other prisons, I finally regained a little strength and my hair grew back. I occupied a cell near where two Tibetan guards were lodged: Nyima, who had been a monk in the monastery of Drepoung and who was authoritarian and cruel, and Tsamla, a young woman who was a decent person. Under the supervision of some Chinese, the couple were responsible for our surveillance. The old-timers from Chonjuk were with me. In the morning when I went to the latrines I could exchange a few words with them. We had to exercise extreme caution because there were always zealous prisoners among us ready to denounce a cell mate.

It was at this period that I made the acquaintance of a lama from Drepoung. In 1959 he had gone to study in China and had abandoned his monastic vows to live with the servant of a woman who sold butter near the monastery. For a long time the couple appeared to be collaborating with the occupation. One day, however, the wife announced a desire to rejoin the Dalai Lama in India. The lama was thrilled by this initiative. The couple and their child left Lhasa secretly to go to Gyantse where they had a relative. From there they planned to reach Bhutan. Unfortunately, soon after their departure soldiers arrested them. The lama was separated from his wife and child and was taken to Drapchi. He became my source of information on the situation in Tibet.

He told me the Chinese were massacring wild animals, which were numerous in our country and quite varied in species. They would set up a machine gun on the platform of a truck and fire a steady stream of bullets into the brush. In the beginning the animals, which we Tibetans never hunted, were taken by surprise. As the animals finally came to recognize them, the Chinese sent Tibetans to hunt in their place, armed with old guns that had been abandoned by the Tibetan army in its retreat. The lama also explained to me that the fauna, formerly so rich, was totally disappearing. The occupiers hunted small game, especially the hares that were abundant in the hills, by exploding dynamite sticks. Terrorized, the animals would run down the opposite slope toward the plain, where they threw themselves by the hundreds into outstretched nets. Before this intensive hunting, the wild yaks were equally numerous. Soon only a few male animals were left here and there; all the others had been struck down by machine guns, cut up on the spot and loaded on trucks that brought the meat to the military garrisons. Some of it was transported to China. Thousands of wild donkeys were killed. The soldiers also tracked otters. Their skinned bodies rotted near the rivers. The ibex suffered a veritable carnage near Mount Kalaish at their mating time. Their hides, which were sold in Lhasa and other cities, were used for making warm clothes for the Chinese who especially feared the cold. Ponds, lakes, and streams were red with their blood and soiled with excrement. As the lama knew the particular region well, the military had used him as a guide for a good number of expeditions. It was thus that he came to see the innumerable horns and all the animal skulls that had been abandoned in the valleys.

These accounts revolted me. Several years later they gave me permission to go to Potangmo where, under Chinese surveillance, I was supposed to teach Tibetan doctors how to prepare the precious pills. I saw many posters there advocating protection of the flora and fauna. What lies and hypocrisy! As I moved around I learned that the Chinese collected fledgling birds from their nests and fried them, claiming there was no more tender flesh. One day I saw some monkeys that soldiers had trapped. To capture them the hunters had let loose their dogs to more easily trap them. The poor beasts were torn apart alive. One of the monkeys raised a thumb to the executioners as if asking to be spared. The Chinese thought that was hilarious. They cracked open their skulls to 'savor' the brains that they said were a strong aphrodisiac.

Today a part of our vast territory srves as a depository for nuclear waste; the flora and fauna in these parts have been destroyed. That is of extreme gravity. Everything that was the basis of the Tibetan people's pride, everything that composed the extraordinary richness of our country, that constituted its unique culture, is in the process of disappearing.

Drapchi was a real antechamber of death. The inhabitants of Taktser, the birthplace of His Holiness the Dalai Lama, were imprisoned there. Day and night they howled like beasts. No-one paid any attention to their cries and one day they stopped. We wondered if they had been killed, transferred somewhere else, hospitalized? No-one ever found out. Anything was possible at Drapchi. In a cell near mine there was a prisoner from Nyemo who attempted an escape. It must have been four o'clock in the morning. We heard shouts, machine-gun fire, and the thud of a body falling. The man was carried to the hospital where he died from his wounds. In another cell a prisoner hanged himself. He had torn up his blanket and made a rope with it. They found him in the early morning hours. It was amazing that these deaths were covered up in Drapchi.

At night my prayers were often interrupted by the cries of Tibetan women who were being tortured. Sometimes they endured these atrocities for nothing more than stealing a few vegetables from a garden. They risked dying at Drapchi because they were hungry and their children were wasting away. Death must have seemed almost sweet to them because first they were raped and then beaten. I had heard that one of the female Tibetan guards was particularly cruel toward her sisters. I could never understand why. I suffered for these women and I prayed for them, for all of us.

I wondered what became of the prisoners' bodies. Persistent rumors circulated in Drapchi and in the other camps at Lhasa. It was a long time before we understood why prisoners often refused to be operated on in the hospital. I heard about a young girl who came to the hospital to visit her father and bring him a little sack of *tsampa*. She was told by the guards that he was suffering from an inoperable tumor in his stomach and had been transferred to the Chinese hospital in Lhasa. His family believed the Chinese had done everything in their power to care for him. In reality they had killed the man and removed his organs to sell them. Such occurrences multiplied and fear settled in at Drapchi. At the time doctors were supposedly coming from China especially to operate on Tibetans, who were said to have a tendency to fall ill suddenly and die. It was also at this time that I had confirmation that forced abortions were being performed. Before 1959, I had already heard about this from people from the occupied regions of Kham and Amdo.

Three years went by and then one morning a Tibetan guard ordered me to gather my things. I was transferred by truck with some others to the Taksoung Khang prison, to continue my 're-education'. It was May 1965 (the year serpent-wood). That year the question of Tibet was again discussed at the United Nations at the request of Thailand, the Philippines, Malta, Ireland, Melanesia, Nicaragua, and El Salvador, all countries that I had never heard of. The Indian contingency also voted in favor of the resolution. But we knew nothing of all that in prison. The only information that reached us from Dharamsala, where our government in exile was installed and where the Dalai Lama lived, came from the new arrivals. Thus I learned that His Holiness was doing everything he could to open the eyes of the world to the fate of the Tibetan people.

Taksoung Khang consisted of three hills, in the middle of which rose the prison. As the weeks went by I noticed that most of the prisoners were in the same situation as I. None of them had been officially sentenced. For the first time I met Tibetan resistors; they had been trained in Arizona by the CIA and then parachuted into Tibet. It was rare that they let themselves be taken alive. These men of exemplary courage preferred death to capture and did not hesitate to bite into the cyanide capsule they all carried.

Very quickly I understood the reasons for this sudden

transfer to Taksoung Khang. For the Chinese authorities my situation was far from clear because I still refused to deny the Dalai Lama and his family. The *thamzing* sessions resumed on a daily basis. This time my tormentors' invectives were directed at His Holiness. As they would not let up, I finally said to them: 'I have committed no crime against your country. I have never been a spy. If you believe that I have done bad things, then execute me. I am not afraid and I am not uneasy about my death.'

I occupied cell number 5. Every day I received a visit from a Tibetan who questioned me on the reasons for my transfer to Taksoung Khang. I was mistrustful and for good reason. This man was a collaborator and he was there only to extract information from me about my relations with the Yapchi family. He wanted me to tell him how I managed to get my information to Gyelo Dhondup, the Dalai Lama's brother, who was then in India at Kalimpong.

Every afternoon there was enforced reading of propaganda newspapers. Knowing I was going to be questioned on the material, I retained a few ideas and then spent the rest of my time reciting mantras. I felt a growing pressure on me. The prisoners were now being transferred from one camp to another. Surveillance had been tightened and it was becoming more difficult to make contact with anyone. It was only when I went to the latrine for my needs that I could exchange a few brief words.

In 1966 (the year horse-fire) the Red Guards made their appearance at Lhasa. China was enforcing the Cultural Revolution and the situation in our country worsened. The spirit of resistance caught fire again among the Tibetans, and predictably there were daily reprisals of repression, murder, and pillaging by the Chinese occupiers.

At Taksoung Khang I met a man named Lobsang who spoke to me about a trip he had made to India and he related a vision he had of two blackbirds flying from Tibet to India. For Tibetans, the blackbird is an emanation of Mahakala, one of the most important protecting deities, to whom a sanctuary is consecrated in almost every temple. I do not know if Lobsang's story was true but it gave me great joy. He also spoke to me about the help that the Tibetan refugees and the government in exile were receiving, and about the vast reconstruction program that the Chinese had put in place in our country.

In prison they kept telling us that Tibetans had entered the modern era. However, this was not really happening. After the Dalai Lama's departure into exile, the Chinese authorities undertook 'democratic reforms', confiscating lands and possessions in order to, as they said, redistribute them to the disadvantaged classes. They proceeded to arrest the so-called enemies of the people, that is, the landowners, the rich, and the reactionaries whom they gradually eliminated in the camps or simply executed on the spot. Communes and agricultural co-operatives were established. But the objectives could never be achieved. One day a saying appeared and spread throughout the country: 'First the Chinese made us laugh, now they make us weep . . .'

In 1962 centers of agricultural experimentation were installed in Lhasa, Chigatse and Lhokha, supported by propaganda vaunting their virtues. The authorities wanted the peasants of the poor classes to see the possibility of a better life, on condition, of course, that they denounce the 'reactionaries'. The Chinese trained 'leaders' in these communes who were then sent into other regions of Tibet to replicate the system. Not content with these 'democratic reforms', the Chinese imposed a rationing system on the peasants: about fifteen kilos of food per person per month. These quotas did not take into account the share of old people or those who were unable to work. By comparison, before 1959, the Tibetan farmers had enough butter, vegetables and meat to feed all the members of their family, young and old.

The nomads, who represented the great majority of the Tibetan population, were forced into settlements. The yaks perished, and famine threatened. Lobsang told me that children in Lhasa were reduced to scavenging in garbage bins and eating the food scraps that the soldiers threw to the pigs. Tibetan women sold their blood to feed their families.

With the Cultural Revolution our daily life in the prison became drastically more harsh. We were awakened at six o'clock. First we lined up at the latrines which we then had to clean. We were given a bowl of tea and a little *tsampa*. Butter tea had become a privilege of the past. From now on the Tibetans would have to be satisfied with black salted tea. The rations were reduced and hunger gnawed at us continuously. One day I learned that Dayul, one of my other sources of information, had been executed. He had eaten an egg and carelessly hid the shells under his thin mattress. A guard found them during a search. He was tortured for a long time before he was killed. Such things are so hard to believe, yet they happened over and over.

I knew another man at Taksoung Khang who had been imprisoned for protesting in 1964 against the arrest of the Panchen Lama. The guards gave him no food at all. He wept night and day but no-one paid any attention to him. At the end, pus ran from his ears and nose. Another prisoner and I were charged with burying his body. Before we covered him with dirt, the guards laughed and pointed at us: 'Take a good look. You'll be like him soon if you keep resisting.' Another of my acquaintances had known the Panchen Lama well and he suffered the same fate: torture and starvation. In his cell he made little balls of his own excrement and swallowed them. Week after week they tortured him and tossed him onto his mattress, his body covered with open wounds and bruises from the beatings.

'The best remedy for a fool is to beat him,' our Chinese as well as our Tibetan jailers would say.

They distributed brochures to us proclaiming the merits of the Cultural Revolution and the new policies of President Mao. The Tibetans were now fully aware of the magnitude of the evil that had swept their country. Religious texts were burned, the effigies and statues that were not carried off to China were thrown into the rivers. Communist propaganda insinuated itself everywhere. A new society had been founded, so the cant went, based on a new ideology, new values, a new culture. All of these innovations, needless to say, were as far from our traditions as from our needs.

Orders were given one day for the prisoners to be totally isolated from the outside. We could no longer have visitors. Information reached us that barricades and barbed wire had been put up around the prison because an uprising of the populace was feared. A few months later, the situation having stabilized somewhat, I was among the prisoners who had to dismantle them. I learned then that practically all the monasteries in Tibet had been sacked, pillaged, and destroyed by the Red Guards. That same evening I thought about the monks at Chothey. I had difficulty sleeping and when I finally did fall asleep I had a strange dream. I was a novice seated above the passageway that led to the garden. With my legs dangling in the void, I was watching my tutor, who was carefully picking apricots. Suddenly an eagle appeared on the horizon, flying toward Chothey. It soared over the garden swooped down and snatched up its prey, a serpent that was about to strike my tutor. Its talons grasped the reptile, crushed its skull, then with a majestic beating of its wings it soared back up, bearing its prey. The image of *Amala* appeared and she was smiling at me. That night I was surprised to find myself crying. It had been so many years since I had had a clear vision of my mother. I felt this was a good omen.

Tibetan children were being enrolled in a sort of institution where they were being taught the thoughts of Mao Zedong and instructed in fabricating light weapons, such as lances and hatchets. The Red Guards distributed these to the young Tibetans so they could help destroy the vestiges of their own past. Misfortune befell the adult who tried to intervene or object. One day a child of about ten refused to destroy a statue of Tara. He described his act of courage to his mother, who was pleased and congratulated him. When the Chinese learned of this young Tibetan's behavior, the mother was publicly humiliated. Some children did try to salvage religious objects from the monasteries around Lhasa, almost all of which had been destroyed. Red

Guards invariably surprised them and under fierce questioning tried to force them to accuse their friends.

Many inhabitants of the region of Nyemo, from which I came, were imprisoned during the Cultural Revolution. There were about thirty of them at Taksoung Khang, easily identifiable by the white *chupa* they wore. One day I noticed a bird with a flat head and yellow eyes that was seeking shelter in the vicinity of my compatriots from Nyemo. The bird was making unusual sounds. This was a bad omen. The next morning there was a commotion. Armed soldiers shouting orders had entered the courtyard. Doors banged open. The noise was coming from the cells occupied by the people from Nyemo. They were handcuffed and led outside where a truck was waiting for them. That evening I learned from the Tibetans who worked in the kitchens that thirty-two compatriots had been executed near Drapchi. From the truck the Nyemos had shouted, 'Long live a free Tibet!' 'Long live Kundun!' 'Free Tibet!' On the place of their execution the soldiers made them dig a ditch, then ordered them to kneel next to it. The Chinese fired on them, each receiving a bullet in the neck. Their bodies were hastily covered with dirt, without anyone checking whether one of them might still be alive. The following week I read in the prison paper that the counter-revolutionaries from Nyemo had been executed. I read, too, that Red Guards had killed some other Tibetans by driving nails into their skulls with hammers.

One day I was pulled from my cell. They told me I would see with my own eyes the changes that had taken place in Tibetan society. I was put in a truck with sixteen other prisoners and taken to a place three hours from Lhasa. I still clearly remember a Tibetan woman who praised the Communist system to us. She told us about the abundance of grains and showed us an enormous stockpile of wheat near the platform where we were standing. I suspected that the whole business must be a show put on for us by the Chinese. The woman shocked me especially when she criticized the government of the Dalai Lama and the former feudal regime, alleging that it was unjust and that exploitation and brutality had been rife. She walked us to an orchard, talking all the while about the dreadful situation that supposedly existed in Tibet before 1959. We were shown a house that had belonged to a rich family of the aristocracy and which, according to her, had been transformed into a school. I did see a few children who were hanging about, but they were in rags. The deception was too crude and I assumed this was just for show.

On our return to Taksoung Khang the Chinese asked if we had been able to perceive the positive evolution in the life of Tibetans.

'Did you notice how the men and women have become perfectly educated and well-informed on the motherland? They're not stubborn like you, who persist in banging your heads against a wall.'

The next day they took us to an exhibition of photography and sculpture that illustrated the backward and barbaric aspects of Tibetan society before 1959. In this hall I saw a clay figurine that represented a monk tearing the eyes out of a little child. In a photograph a Tibetan officer was whipping one of his soldiers. There was also a model of a Tibetan prison, with little figures of prisoners that had no arms. This was supposed to represent the crimes of the Panchen Lama, who according to the Chinese had the hands of many Tibetans cut off before he himself was arrested. In the evening I invoked the divinities' protection of the Panchen Rinpoche.

14

Survival at Yititok

One morning in 1971 (the year pig-iron) several of us were led into a room to finally receive our sentences. Twelve terrible years had passed since my arrest in 1959. I remember that standing there with me were Ouangtchen Gyatok, Ouangdul and Nampeu Pola, all of whom had heavy penalties inflicted on them: Ouangtchen Gyatok was sent to the mechanics section of Yititok prison, Ouangdul to the carpentry section, and Nampeu Pola to the quarry, the harshest and most feared destination. When my turn came an officer read me a letter listing the accusations against me: my trip to Kalimpong, my relations with Gyelo Dhondup, the Dalai Lama's brother, and of course with His Holiness. They also said I had taken part in a vast signature campaign in 1959 to denounce the Chinese presence in Tibet. Finally the sentence fell.

'Seventeen years imprisonment!'

The words seemed to come from far away. The mantra *Om Mani Padme Hum* rang in my head. Seventeen years! I had already survived twelve years! A few days later I was transferred to Yititok where I would join Nampeu Pola. Too old to cut stones, he was assigned to sweeping the kitchen and cleaning vegetables, but every day he was tortured as soon as he was returned to his cell. He tried to commit suicide by cutting off his penis. Chained, beaten with a stick and given electric shocks, he soon died.

At Yititok there were many cells and we were assigned work by sections. The prisoners looked like skeletons and reminded me of those at the Jiuzhen camp in China, where, in three years, seven hundred of eight hundred prisoners had died of exhaustion.

To keep the prisoners from fraternizing the Chinese frequently rotated us. There were usually seven of us in a narrow, dimly lit room. We were ordered to question each other, make reports and be ready to accuse our companions at the *thamzing* sessions. In the evening some of the prisoners would wrap their blanket around their heads to pray. Informers would discreetly draw near to listen to their words in hope of being able to denounce them for something later. When we left our cells we were forbidden to look at another prisoner, much less smile or exchange glances. If we did we were immediately accused of sympathizing with the reactionaries in the pay of the renegade Dalai Lama. When we lined up in the morning for our tea, only then could we murmur a few words in the ear of the person ahead of us, hoping he would not report our remarks to the guards.

At Yititok there were also common-law prisoners who enjoyed a more flexible regime. They generally worked in the prison, in the carpentry section making doors, window frames and beds, and in the mechanic section repairing military vehicles. They worked inside a barbed-wire enclosure guarded by soldiers. When workers were needed in Lhasa they got them from the camp. Carpenters and mechanics would go out in little groups and would be lodged during their four-or-five-month stint in tents near the work site encircled by barbed wire and spikes.

Even though my sentence had been pronounced, the Chinese continued to express suspicion about me, which was why I had been assigned to the quarry. As I have said, this was the most arduous and dangerous assignment. It took us fifteen minutes of painful walking to reach the quarry. We would proceed single file in chains to the foot of the mountain, carrying heavy sacks of tools that hurt our backs. Only the Tibetans did this kind of forced labor; the Chinese prisoners were assigned to other sections. Here in Yititok the chances of surviving slave labor in the quarry were infinitesimal.

The interrogations went on daily. I was soon reduced to a robot state. It reminded me of the Jiuzhen prison but this time I did not imagine I would get out alive. Our jailers beat us with electric truncheons, jabbing them into the mouth, the anus, or placing them on the genitals. In the end, we did not even have the strength to yell. In a permanent state of semi-consciousness, we were nevertheless always aware of the guards' mocking laughter.

The quarry was situated in a valley and was surrounded by wild mountains. We would hear dynamite explosions throughout the day followed by the shattering of rock. The mountain was being stripped. We were divided into groups of six. Two of us worked at extracting the blocks, two others hewed them and the other two shaped them. Producing ninety pieces a day could only be done by working in a team. At the end of each month the Chinese tallied the production. There was no problem when the monthly quota was exceeded, but if we were short we were beaten and told we were bad Communists. We called these treatments the 'vicious cycle of death and rebirth', for the simple reason that if we did not die during the night we would have to go off to the quarry the next morning to break up more rocks.

At the end of several days of this regime our clothes were in tatters. We had no rope and nothing to protect our backs. When clients of the prison brought in flat tires, we would rush to make off with them. The rubber cut up in squares served as protection; if there was an inner tube, we fashioned gloves. We could sometimes cut out large bands that we placed on our backs when we carried the stones. In each team one of the prisoners was put in charge and had to pace the group and denounce them if they slowed down. At the end of the month a list of the work groups by order of their productivity was posted. The ones at the bottom of the list were publicly humiliated.

The first six months of this routine were very painful. My hands were raw. The blisters bled all the time and the skin never healed. The rubber protected us but it did not let in air. In the summer, our clothes and our shoes were so flimsy that we were finally walking barefoot; our clothes were so filthy that they provoked infections in our wounds. Little by little, we learned how to manipulate the tools. The older ones had taught me a technique for driving enormous nails into the grooves of the stones. If we misjudged our hammer blows, rock splinters could rebound as projectiles and penetrate our bodies. If the knees were injured, that was the end.

The pace was so intense in the quarry that many of the prisoners developed cardiac problems. Malnutrition and the repeated effort provoked heart attacks. In the evening after the *thamzing*, we had to help our companions stretch out and breathe, watching that they did not swallow their tongues. Our legs swelled so badly that some of us could not even bend them. Some died on the spot in the quarry, the body suffocated under too heavy a load and the heart gave out. Because the prisoners who worked the quarry dropped like flies, the guards separated us from the other prisoners on the pretext that we were contagious.

The prisoners assigned to the quarry duty at Yititok would admit to any fault, including those they never committed. But the guards continued to strike them on the pretext that they were lying to lighten their sentence. They were most often transferred to the hospital in a coma. As soon as they regained consciousness, the doctors reprimanded them. Returned to the camp, the atrocious torture began all over again. The guards would say to them:

'Chinese doctors are specialists and you can't fool them. You're trying to deceive them. You're lying because you don't want to work for the motherland.'

The blows rained down anew, sometimes the greater part of the day or night. When men died under the torture, their bodies were hastily transported to the hospital.

At the request of the camp authorities Chinese doctors regularly came to examine the corpses and perform experiments, with the avowed aim of studying the heart and brain of Tibetans. Then they would make out a report on the probable cause of death. No-one at Yititok ever died from torture; they died from an illness.

When I prayed I thought more and more about the inevitably nearing moment of my own death. How to survive in such a camp? Even with meditation I had difficulty rallying myself. I grew weaker and weaker and looked like a skeleton, as I had at Jiuzhen. When one of us died we would divide up his clothes. But others died themselves before they had a chance to put the clothes on. The dead were buried in ditches near the monastery of Sera or near Drapchi prison.

On Sundays the jailers distributed needles and thread so we could repair our rags. The basic piece of clothing was usually black, but we added to it all sorts of colored cloth scraps that we found, pieces from tires and even shoe soles. When we lacked enough thread we would collect the guards' worn gloves and take them apart patiently thread by thread.

Every day before going back into our cells we had to line up facing the guards, still with the iron toolbox on our backs. They would give us a bowl of tea. Then for one, two, sometimes three hours, we praised President Mao. We would also sing:

'We have Communist China as our guide. We study and we learn the ideology, according to the wishes of Mao.'

One evening a monk who had just received a beating was supposed to join us in our 'singing'. He could barely stand. Suddenly, as a truck crossed the prison yard, he bolted from the ranks and threw himself under the wheels and died instantly. Suicides like this occurred daily at Yititok. The same thing was happening outside the prisons. I heard that Tibetans, both men and women, would prostrate themselves three times before the Potala and then throw themselves into the Kyitchou river.

One day in 1972 (the year mouse-water) my cell door opened to admit an unusual monk. His name was Pelden Gyatso and he had already racked up three long years in the Chinese prisons. For a long time he had occupied a cell three down from mine and we had been able to exchange a few words. But it was only after his transfer into my cell that we got to know and appreciate each other. In the evenings following his arrival, Pelden Gyatso described what he had lived through during twenty months of hospitalization for cardiac problems. When a patient died, they would open the body to find out the cause of death and, especially, to see if the heart, liver, and kidneys were undamaged. If so, they were removed and sent to China to be sold. The Chinese used hermetically sealed boxes which held several glass containers in which the organs were placed. When the dead person's condition was too poor, the body was dissected and used for the instruction of young doctors. Pelden Gyatso especially remembered a young man named Trinle, who died in the hospital. He was dissected by a Chinese woman who removed his heart. If a patient recovered, the doctors could boast about the quality of their care. But if they needed organs, a life counted for little. A dead body was still useful to them and profitable.

When Pelden Gyatso was suffering, I would immediately come to his aid. When my morale was low or I was seriously injured, he helped me. He would ask me to pray with him to the protecting deities. One day we were both designated to work on the construction of an electrical generator on the heights of Lhasa. We were living in a tent and during the day we had a few moments' rest when we could wash our clothes. Pelden Gyatso told me he had no soap and I said I would prepare some for him and that we needed to gather up ashes and collect water from the stream. When the clothes were washed with the mixture they were as clean as if real soap had been used. I also taught him the use of certain roots and a few plants to better resist infections.

I never thought I would meet another person to whom I could express all my suffering. I believe it was the same for him. We found refuge in the Dharma which helped us endure the torture, the moral and physical wounds, and the hunger. Pelden Gyatso and I became very close. As soon as we felt a danger threatening one of us, our senses were on alert. One morning at the quarry I did not feel well. The day before we had endured a heavy *thamzing* session. Pelden Gyatso had been horribly beaten and I was attacked, although less severely. In neighboring cells, Tibetans had died during the night and their bodies had immediately been carried off by the guards. That day I was cutting an enormous stone when it broke in two. In panic, I sidestepped, but a chip pierced my foot. Instantly I felt violent pain as the blood gushed from the wound. My heart was beating wildly. I was afraid because for some time now I had been experiencing heart problems. They were less serious than in other prisoners, but with this wound anything could happen. Some prisoners surrounded me. Pelden Gyatso helped to hoist me into a cart and then I lost consciousness. When I came to I was in my cell and my wound had been bandaged.

The next day I was back working in the quarry. My heart had withstood the shock but I had lost a lot of blood. Fortunately I was able to find some roots with curative properties. In the evening I asked a Tibetan guard for authorization to prepare a moxibustion treatment for myself and he agreed. Blisters had appeared on my foot and the moxibustion would absorb the liquid from them. Barely able to put my foot on the ground, I had suffered greatly all day long. I first took my pulse to ascertain whether I had a fever because if that were the case, I could not intervene in this manner. I lacked the proper instruments and had to use what I could find, a piece of heavy paper of poor quality made from horse manure and the needles we used for sewing our ragged clothes. I made a fire and then planted the heated needles into four specific points around the wound. I applied the paper, impregnated with garlic to permit adhesion, to my foot. Some time later the wound closed and I could walk normally again.

To be treated at the prison hospital the wounded and the sick had to queue up. We waited to be called by the assistant of the doctor, who was a pro-Chinese Tibetan. One day two prisoners who were waiting to be seen were talking about the recent events in Lhasa that they had read about in a newspaper distributed in the cells. The assistant surprised them in their conversation and reported them to the guards. Chained up, they were forced to admit their errors, most notably of criticizing Chinese policy in Tibet. In the days that followed this incident other prisoners wre tortured and four Tibetans committed suicide by cutting their own throats with their quarry tools.

*   *   *

The Cultural Revolution continued to deal severely with Tibet. There were many reasons for the Tibetan people to rebel. The authorities violently put down revolts, despatching special forces into the most zealous regions. Tens of thousands of Tibetans had died in the camps. Humiliated, wasted, annihilated, some actually even thanked their torturers. Once freed, they said they remained grateful to them for the atrocities and the humiliations they had endured. Outside, in the cities and villages, my compatriots endured constant government intrusion: house searches, required declarations of pregnancy, forced contraception. The policy of controlling births continues to this day and reports reveal that, since 1960, girls who had been sterilized and pregnant women were used as guinea pigs for unscrupulous Chinese 'scientists'. In submitting to the demands of the Chinese administration, the Tibetan woman lost all her rights, including the right of control over her own body. From the instant of conception, the Tibetan child was appropriated by the Chinese state, which handed him a birth certificate like a deed of ownership. Daily the authorities exercised their right to kill children and women whose only crime was to be born or give birth without the authorization of the occupying administration.

The Chinese Communists wanted to eradicate our civilization completely. The Red Guards destroyed everything that was even remotely connected to the Tibetan culture. Monastic robes were made into *chupas* for women, religious headpieces were torn into strips from which they made shoes. When they did not simply make off with them, they ground up turquoise stones under the eyes of the wealthy families and threw them to the winds. When they went after the families of the nobility, the Chinese forced the men into *thamzing* sessions during which they placed a red-hot iron bar on their shoulders. I was told again and again that to escape these tortures many Tibetans drowned themselves in the river. At Yititok the guards were fond of a particular form of torture: they attached receptacles around the prisoners' necks containing human urine and excrement and forced them to lower their heads into it and remain like that for hours.

In spite of the searches, some Tibetans managed to hide statues and effigies of the Buddha, sometimes precious stones. One day in the quarry, when I was getting ready to cut an enormous block of stone, I noticed another one, smaller and square. There was no guard near me. I picked it up and saw that it had already been cut. I broke it open and found a small package containing a necklace with a silver amulet decorated with false turquoise and coral stones. The object had no value and must have belonged to a very poor woman. In panic, she had perhaps hidden here the few things she still possessed.

Our people tried to apply the Dharma and this drew down the wrath of the occupiers. 'The Dharma is our patrimony,' we would often repeat. 'We will have lost all when black serpents slither on the ground.' The black serpent so much resembled the long convoy of Chinese trucks winding its way around the bends on the wide roads of the Tibetan plateaus. Despite the repression, the Tibetans continued to affirm: 'We should carry a *mala* in one hand and a prayer wheel in the other and recite continuously the mantra *Om Mani Padme Hum* because we are all the children of Chenrezik.' I learned also that some Tibetan women appeared to be very co-operative with the soldiers, serving them tea or a meal, but this was often to be better able to smash their skulls with an ax blow when the opportunity presented itself. They would, of course, be immediately imprisoned in Drapchi, where most of them died.

At the end of 1972, all the able prisoners of Yititok were gathered and taken to Drapchi, where more than five hundred detainees took part in a special *thamzing* session. For the occasion, they told us to wear Mao's Little Red Book around our necks. The day before we had to wash our tattered clothes. At Drapchi a platform had been hastily constructed. Posters denouncing separatist activities were everywhere. The military personnel watched us, stationed behind heavy machine guns that were kept trained on us. An officer was the first to speak. He insisted on the need to clean Tibet of all the counter-revolutionaries in the pay of the Dalai Lama. He also announced that two prisoners had tried to escape and in the course of their interrogation had admitted their errors. That was a pure lie! We all knew that the two men confessed to none of the crimes that had been imputed to them. Now in chains on the platform, their bodies swollen from beatings, they had to listen to the verdict that condemned them to be executed for offending the popular government. The Chinese had composed a song just for them. I no longer remember the exact words, but it went something like this:

If you kill a separatist,
That's only one.

If you kill two of them,
That's only two.
If you kill three of them,
That's still only three . . .
Only by eliminating all the separatists
Do you get lasting satisfaction.

The prisoners were forced to take up this song as the two men were put in a truck that immediately rumbled off. A few minutes later, before the common ditch situated behind Drapchi, they were executed with a bullet in the back of the neck. The soldiers then fired three more bullets into the bodies.

The patent failure of the Cultural Revolution forced Mao to pass the torch to Chou en Lai. The party leadership was riddled with men devoted to radical propositions. In Tibet the situation hardly changed. At the beginning of 1973 (the year cattle-water) Tibetan guards were made to give their self-criticism before the prisoners. New 'leaders' were named. We were astonished at this sudden reversal but for all that the camps did not empty out and the tortures continued.

It was at this period that I received a visit in my cell from several Chinese officers who wanted to ask me to diagnose and treat their illnesses. The first was a commander of an artillery unit. I asked why he had this sudden interest in Tibetan medicine and he explained that all the other treatments he had tried had failed. It was his last recourse. I took his pulse and prescribed a medication that he could obtain at Men-Tsee-Khang. Then there was a soldier who was suffering from epileptic seizures. I prescribed moxibustions and he was better after a few weeks. One day, it was a

Tibetan prisoner, Nyima Tachi, who received authorization to consult me. He was supposed to go cut down
trees. I advised against it but he was hardly able to
follow my advice. The truck that picked him up with his
work unit overturned and the occupants were injured.
Nyima Tachi was struck in the head by a wheel and
died in the hospital. I learned later that while en route
the men had heard the lowing of a yak but that there
was no herd in the immediate area. This was, in fact, a
bad omen.

Months passed. If the Chinese were to be believed, I
was almost at the end of my sentence. Seventeen years
in the prisons and the camps had not dimmed my hope
of one day seeing the Dalai Lama and his entourage
again. I should have been freed in March 1976 (the year
dragon-fire). In 1974 (the year tiger-wood) I was still
cutting stones in the quarries around Yititok. From time
to time in the evenings I would receive a visit in my
cell. One day the wife of a functionary of Taksoung
Khang, who was temporarily in China, asked me for a
consultation. When I took her pulse, I realized that her
condition was extremely critical and that she probably
had no more than two or three months to live. I advised
her to telephone her husband immediately and to enter
the military hospital of Sera where Chinese doctors
would quickly take charge of her. The woman had an
operation and lived only another month. The surgeons
who operated on her learned about her visit to Yititok,
but were totally misinformed about my diagnosis,
believing that I had estimated she would live another
three or four years. They told me later that she would
probably still be alive if they had been aware of my
diagnosis.

One day the artillery commander came back. This time, he was with the official in charge of the dispensary at Yititok, Dr Li, who had a cynical attitude toward me. I supposed he had come to test me. I presented my diagnosis to him. The doctor, standing near him, did not say a word. Then he took the officer's place and held out his arm to me. I took his pulse and, after a little time, I told him he was suffering from a serious liver problem, but that there was in Tibetan medicine, an excellent treatment for this illness. He confirmed to me the exactness of the diagnosis and acknowledged that no Chinese medicine had succeeded in curing him and that he had been told his illness was chronic. I wrote out a prescription on a simple piece of paper. Despite the fact that he was considered incurable, the treatment rapidly gave him positive results.

When I had to treat the artillery commander, I did not forget my prisoner status. I had a strong intuitive sense, like a signal: I absolutely must cure this man. I feel I performed my work with this patient with devotion and sincerity, but I was also fully aware that the Chinese were testing me and, if they were satisfied, I might be allowed to assuage the suffering of many of the prisoners. One of the required qualities of the doctor is the desire to come to the aid of another. Our feeling of concern about the well-being of others – of all others – may also be called compassion. Dispensed impartially, it transcends all barriers and knows no borders. Whether one cares for a friend or an enemy, it is a question of absence of prejudice. Friend or enemy, the doctor must treat all patients exactly the same: they are people who are suffering. Thus he is able to extend his love and kindness to his enemy. When animated by compassion, this sense of responsibility with regard to others, we may truly modify the nature of things and of our actions.

This is how I began to care for patients at Yititok. I had already spent more than sixteen years in the Chinese prisons and I had succeeded in surviving.

Part Three

1976–1998

15

Caring for One's Enemies

The end of 1975 (the year hare-wood) was near. I
had not been working in the quarry for several weeks
now. The Chinese authorities wanted me to pursue
my doctoring activities inside the camp. High-ranking
military people and important officials of the Autonomous Region continued to consult me. The guards had
also gotten into the habit of coming to see me at the
hospital, where I was watched by Chinese nurses. And
Dr Li had authorized me to help care for the prisoners. I
felt sad and powerless because their conditions for the
most part were serious. Assisted by Seupa, a Tibetan
with whom I was going to share my last years in prison,
I could not do much for them but I would try to stay
with them to the end.

Theoretically, I had completed my sentence but
no-one mentioned the possibility of my release. I talked
to Li about it, who advised patience because there
was serious discussion about opening a Tibetan medical
center and I would have my place there. On 22 March,
1976 (the year dragon-fire), I was transferred at Dr Li's
request to Outridu. This was a section of the prison
where they usually placed the prisoners who were at

the end of their sentences or those who had been granted a partial release. It had been built a few months earlier by the prisoners of Yititok. The entrance to Outridu was to the west of the camp and just two steps from the hospital. To the left of the entrance were four buildings where the guards and the security personnel were lodged.

The hospital had a few rooms, a waiting room and a dirty room used for giving injections. I went there to see my patients every morning. Sixty to eighty people would be lined up in the little room that I occupied: prisoners, guards, Chinese military and even sick people from the immediate area who paid a yuan for the consultation. As I had no access to medicines, I gave them a prescription that they could have filled at Men-Tsee-Khang, which might also perfectly well refuse to give it to them.

One day Dr Li came to see me. He was beaming. He told me he was cured and he praised me effusively, complimenting my sincerity and honesty. I was particularly pleased. He promised to submit a request to speed up my release and make it possible for me to practice medicine in Lhasa. I answered that I did my best to treat all the patients, regardless of who they were. In prison, I had developed my capacity to forgive. I said to him that it is only by love and compassion that one can lead one's worst enemy to change his mind.

My life was strewn with innumerable obstacles but I also aspired to happiness and I knew that it would grow as my freedom grew. Free, I would be able to rejoin the Dalai Lama and the Yapchi family. Free, I could go to my birth village, near Nyemo, and to the Chothey monastery. *Lossar*, the celebration of the new year dragon-fire (1976) had just ended when Li informed me of new plans of the Chinese authorities: the opening of a modern hospital at Yititok. I reminded him that I had reached the end of my sentence and that after seventeen years of forced labor, I aspired to recover not only my complete freedom but also my status as a doctor. I reminded him as well that we lacked medicines at Yititok and needed to import plants from India, Nepal, or parts of China for certain remedies. Soon after I received authorization to leave Yititok to collect some medicinal substances. They also provided me with electrical filtering and grinding machines to be used in the preparation of medicines. Dr Li also arranged that on my first outing I could go to Men-Tsee-Khang.

Freedom, I already felt its reflection in Li's behavior toward me and that of the several Chinese officers whom I had treated. On the twenty-second day of the third month of the year dragon-fire, after seventeen years of incarceration, I left the prison as an almost free man. When I crossed the threshold I felt an immense relief. Of course I would have been happier if things had been different on the outside and the lives of Tibetans had really changed, as the Communist propaganda claimed. But this was not the case. The Red Guards and the Cultural Revolution, with its insane excesses, had taken their toll. The people of Lhasa walked about haggard, their eyes cast down. Their legendary smile had disappeared. Mostly they looked away when they saw me. It is true that I wore a head covering that marked my prisoner status, which could put people on their guard. Fear could be read in people's expressions and in their bearing. I respected them, taking care not to put them in danger, because a simple gesture might have been enough to overturn their lives.

The Tibetans' happiness had been destroyed and now seemed unattainable. As a doctor I can verify that a person whose mind is peaceful also feels well and his body is in balance. The person who has a troubled mind will see his health deteriorate. If the Chinese had behaved differently toward us, perhaps we might have followed them and shared certain economic and social concepts, even political. There are many good things in the original ideals of Marxism; but certainly not this totalitarianism or this corrupt form of Communism that is practiced in China, against which we must whole-heartedly continue to fight.

I saw children, six or seven years old, picking through pig troughs. Nowhere did I rediscover the scent of incense. With an uncertain step I went to Men-Tsee-Khang. My master, Khenrab Norbu, had died in 1962 (the year tiger-water). The place did not seem unfamiliar to me when I arrived. The institute had not developed and there were few new buildings. The houses around Men-Tsee-Khang had evidently been damaged and looted and were being rebuilt, but I did not encounter a single one of the original occupants and I saw only a few people whom I knew. They avoided me or were hesitant, and when they finally spoke to me it was to warn me against the Chinese! In Lhasa the Chinese had nicknamed me the 'dissident doctor'. Those who knew me well were shocked, for that could also be interpreted to mean that I was getting rich off the backs of my compatriots. An absurd idea, but it was what the Chinese wanted people to believe about the Dalai Lama and those close to him. Friends said to me: 'It is unjust. You are not such a man, you are still *Lhamenpa*, and you have kept your integrity.'

'You are perfectly right.' I answered them. 'I have never broken any law. In the eyes of the Chinese, my only wrong is having been the doctor of Kundun and his mother. It's the Chinese who have introduced this notion of dissidence but we Tibetans have no reason to use it.'

At Men-Tsee-Khang I was received with understandable mistrust. I was the 'spy in semi-liberty' and the students there were doubtless indebted to the Communist Chinese. I presented myself to a professor. Suddenly the image of Khenrab Norbu surged up in me. There was not the slighest comparison with the person in front of me and I quickly recovered my composure. I hoped only to borrow a medical text. The professor told me I might consult it in the institute but there was no question of taking it with me. I saw only young doctors. All of my professors were dead. I felt a deep sadness, and doubtless a shred of revolt, but I kept quiet: I was a 'dissident'. I had noticed they were building some walls inside the institute and I told myself that the future would perhaps be better. One thing consoled me: there were hardly any Chinese about. In the past they dismissed Tibetan medicine, according to them it had no therapeutic efficacy. Still, they consulted me in prison and a few Chinese spoke up to prevent our medicine and our entire therapeutic arsenal from disappearing. Dr Li was one of these. At the time the precious pills were taken by high-ranking dignitaries of the Communist hierarchy. They were labeled as 'Chinese medicine' but their conception and their mode of preparation were no less Tibetan. Beijing went quite far in its medical propaganda. A Communist text that was translated into Tibetan affirmed that these medicines and procedures had their distant origin in China. The doctors claimed that the pills were prepared by the 'Great Sanctuary of Chinese Medicine' and their utilization would be extended into Tibet. In fact, our principal medical texts had been burned by the Red Guards and China had nearly destroyed what today it was claiming to have created. The occupying authorities had developed medical structures in the principal cities of Tibet using relatively sophisticated material, generally of foreign origin. But all that was, of course, reserved for the Chinese; the Tibetans were excluded except for very special interventions.

One day as I was returning from the hospital I met several Tibetans who had studied with me at Men-Tsee-Khang. Not one of them invited me to take tea. I was stung by this but I also understood their attitude. Our city lived in mistrust, which was infinitely sad and pitiful but also the normal state of affairs these days. Some of my former patients did not hesitate to invite me to their homes in spite of the risks they were running. I took care of them secretly but I was regularly followed. I would leave a house and it would immediately be searched and the family threatened. One day I was even harshly reprimanded by some soldiers who thought I went about too much in Lhasa. The next day, I underwent a *thamzing* session and Dr Li could do nothing for me.

In the course of my visits my compatriots told me what their daily lives had been since the Dalai Lama's exile. A family would prepare tea when they had a little butter but they would have to be careful. A neighbor might smell it and report them. They would be reproached for living an extravagant bourgeois life, for not rejecting the obsolete ways of the past. The Tibetans were living in an atmosphere of mistrust and suspicion. I noticed no change in conditions, even after Mao's death, in September 1976. The soldiers made their rounds every night, searching for potential resisters. As soon as a stranger arrived in a house, they would show up. They searched the house, interrogated the family, demanded to know not only about the visitor's identity, but also about the person's opinions. This 'freedom' under surveillance was a living hell. I noticed also that while the Tibetans worked hard in the fields, the grain they produced was requisitioned by the army. My 'free' countrymen were dying of starvation as fast as those who were incarcerated.

More and more patients came for a consultation at Outridu, but we lacked medicines. Men-Tsee-Khang was unable to furnish us with any and we had an annual budget for this purpose of only five hundred yuan. We could do nothing with this paltry amount. I discussed this with Dr Li, who said that if I knew where to find the plants and minerals, he would organize an expedition. He then obtained all the authorizations to move about sixty prisoners selected by their physical condition and the fact that they were at the end of their sentences. We left the camp under a heavy escort about one o'clock in the morning and reached the mountain at daybreak. Of little importance were the cold and the violent gales of wind that lashed our cheeks and flattened our pants and our *chupas* against our legs.

We advanced in single file, bent over double, with our caps pulled down over our ears. There was no possibility of shelter. Trees were scarce because of the altitude, so there was not much natural protection.

I walked with great difficulty. The Chinese in charge of the group walked on my right; Seupa, a Tibetan doctor who worked with me at Outridu, was on my left. When he saw me stagger a little, he took my arm to hold me up. Seupa was aware of my extreme weakness but he needed me for the harvesting of the plants and the gathering of certain stones.

Suddenly the wind and rain stopped and a double rainbow appeared against the contours of the mountain. It was a good omen and I remarked on it to Seupa, who smiled at me. Looking up, I noticed that on the other side of a stream the bank rose steeply to form an escarpment. I went first through the icy water. It was so good to experience sensations from the past again. That precise instant was a special moment that unfortunately I could not share with anyone. But Dr Seupa was watching me and I believe he read my feelings.

The bank, hollowed by the current, formed an outcropping and sheltered a carpet of roots and shrubbery. I signaled to Li and the group stopped. The soldiers set up a tent while I asked my companions to undo the bags that had been unloaded from the mules. We made a fire. During the night the weather changed again. When at daybreak I went out of the tent, the sun made a gentle appearance. We spent several days gathering plants. I knew of a grotto in the area where we were able to find the stones we had come to look for. Seupa advised me against carrying the sacks but I insisted, wishing to do as much as my companions who were suffering as much as I. Some of them were carrying as much as fifty kilos; I was unable to manage even half that weight.

On returning to Outridu, the sacks were loaded onto a truck for transport to Men-Tsee-Khang, which in exchange for the raw materials would furnish us with the medicines. I could not care for all the patients. Only the most seriously ill received treatment; the others had to wait. This was not without problems. The prisoners, especially, accused me of favoring the outside patients whom they considered collaborators. My explanations no longer satisfied them. Some even complained to the administration. Dr Li had to intervene again, explaining to the local authorities that I took into account only the state of health of my patients and that we lacked medicines.

We made the trip several more times in 1977 (the year serpent-fire). I noticed that the plants had become very scarce in certain areas, especially around Lhasa. We had to cross another valley and continue higher into the mountain. We met nomads, who offered us tea out of sight of the guards. This allowed me a little time for praying and for making a traditional ritual sacrifice: I offered a *kata* and threw it into a fire of juniper branches.

My reputation had grown even more. The Tibetans knew now that they could consult an *amchi* and that I had been Kundun's doctor. The Chinese also came to see me in growing numbers. They allotted me a salary, the sum of thirty yuan, which covered my meager expenses for clothing and food. One of my patients told me that the precious pills were even much valued in Beijing and other large cities in China. He praised my diagnostic ability, my knowledge of Tibetan medicine, and emphasized that I had the opportunity to serve the motherland at the moment when Tibet had become a prosperous country. He quickly changed his tone though and reminded me that the Land of Snows existed in times past in ignorance and under the oppression of a renegade, who wanted to be called the Dalai Lama, and his band. He accused me of having belonged to this 'clan' of bandits.

I answered in a firm tone that I was a simple monk who had just finished his medical studies when the Chinese entered Tibet. 'Everything you say is perhaps true,' I said, 'but I don't see your point.'

'Ah!' he exclaimed. 'You still don't understand . . .'

That evening, having returned to my cell, I invoked Tara to protect me from this man, who had obviously come to try to destroy me, once again. I fell asleep thinking about the monks of Chothey.

Finally, in April 1978 (the year horse-earth) I was given authorization to go to Chothey. As I set out on foot, thin rays of sun announcing the spring filtered through the trees. Shrubs were rather scarce in the undergrowth. A few trees had fallen, others tilted dangerously, victims of heavy snowfalls the previous winter. The forest that I was crossing on the road to Nyemo was noticeably sparse. I had heard from the prisoners that the Chinese practiced an aggressive deforestation. Now I had the proof before my eyes. Trucks, loaded with tree trunks, passed me, raising clouds of dust.

Undecided as to the direction to take, I chose the road that led me toward a pass. The walk warmed me but in the evening, exhausted by so much effort, I shivered in the cold air. I found shelter in a grotto and rolled myself into a ball in the blanket I had brought along. Just as I was now doing in crossing this forest, I had made my way on a difficult twisting path, through obstacles that this human life imposed on me. Since the visit of one of my uncles at Drapchi, I had had no news of my family. He had told me of Pessala's death and of two other uncles in Chinese prisons. Eyes wide open, I watched the darkness fall around me. I tried to light a fire to push back the gloom but the dampness prevented the wood from catching. I heard noises and murmurs and I did not dare move; an animal was foraging in the bushes. It sniffed and then went away. Suddenly, I could not stand it any more and I gave in to my distress. My throat knotted and my body was shaken with heavy sobs. I felt alone, worn out, tired of living through so much suffering. Finally I fell asleep thinking that in two days I would be at Chothey.

In the early hours I was awakened by thirst. I heard the rushing sound of a waterfall and the stream, which I soon saw, was soothing. I drank eagerly to quench my thirst. Hunger was also gnawing at me, but I had no more *tsampa*. I looked for some roots and leaves. The day before I had felt lost in this setting that brought so many old memories back to me. The second day was as painful as the first.

I met some nuns who, in spite of threats, had decided to return to their convent of Gargompa. They told me the Red Guards had totally destroyed their monastery. They were traveling through the region trying to collect donations that would permit them to complete the reconstruction work. There were very few nuns left at Gargompa. Some of the young nuns had been raped by the Chinese, some had fled to Lhasa, where they took part in demonstrations against the occupation. They were very likely arrested and never heard from again. Others had preferred to kill themselves. A few left for India, thanks to the help of people who lived in the area, and they found refuge at Dharamsala. Those who remained at Gargompa had to make out the best they could for clothing and food. They also told me that all the monasteries in the area had been pillaged and most of them torn down. I immediately thought of Chothey and hurried on my way.

I was exhausted by so much effort and my progress became more difficult. Hunger also caused such relentless pain that I was forced to stop and enter into meditation. The warmth that coursed through my body did me much good and calmed me. In the evening I found shelter in the house of an old woman. She happened to have a high fever that I was able to treat. Before leaving the house the next day, I collected some medicinal plants for her. Now only a few hours separated me from Nyemo. That night in the dark I thought I heard an owl but I was not sure. For Tibetans, that would have been a very bad omen.

It was now raining off and on and I found shelter where I could, by a tree or a rock, or in a grotto. But this slowed my progress toward the monastery and I decided to walk a little further. I spent a last night near a lake where I could finally light a fire with some juniper branches. Taking advantage of the fire I burned some incense. In the distance, the low rumble of thunder reverberated on the snowy peaks.

Chothey . . . I stayed still for a long moment, considering the best route to take. My eagerness to reach the monastery made me walk faster. Taking care not to slip, I started to cross the bridge over the river, the last obstacle. I discovered some of the boards were missing and I had to turn back. I found a path that descended into the gorge and I took that. The noise was terrifying. The shock of water beating against the rocks with an unbelievable force awoke in me images of my adolescence. To rejoin the path that ascended from the other bank I had no other choice but to wade through the river. The water was icy and the current violent and I fought not to lose my footing, not to be swept away a hundred meters further on. I gathered all my strength and finally reached the other bank. I climbed the trail, happy not to have to take a long detour.

Ahead of me as far as the eye could see was solitude and silence. Wild flowers carpeted the meadows that led to the monastery. The sun became brighter and dazzled me. Chothey, the monks, my tutor! My heart beat wildly. Was it a vision? The high wall was riddled with dark holes, like immense crevasses, that had not been there before. It had been twenty-five years. So long ago, yet like yesterday. But these gaping holes caused by the explosion of dynamite held my attention. And the silence, suddenly so heavy? A wave of panic unfurled in me. I opened the heavy door to the prayer room onto a vision of horror and destruction!

Everything had been demolished, the statues, the relics, the effigies. I went into a loft. Some restoration work had been undertaken here and there but everything seemed to have been abandoned. The two-story-high representation of the Buddha, in bronze and gold, had been removed and replaced with another smaller statue made of clay. All the gold mural paintings had disappeared.

At that instant, shaken with sobs, I was overcome with despair. When I stopped crying, I was still distraught and did not notice the furtive movements around me. About thirty monks had come forward to greet me. They were all very thin and I had difficulty recognizing my tutor among them. He presented me with a *kata* and tea was offered. I learned that the relics had been taken away, the effigies sold in foreign places, and the sacred texts were somewhere in China. Revolt and anger gnawed at me. Why destroy Chothey, Ganden, Drepoung, Sera, and more than six thousand other temples and monasteries? Why these massive transfers of Chinese people into Tibet? Why all this suffering? Why this destruction? Where was the tolerance, the wisdom preached by the masters of Beijing? My story is dedicated also to the memory of Chothey. I think of my fellow monks. My monastery is still partially destroyed. I hope only that these few thoughts will be able to help in some way all those who still live there. Chothey is in my heart and my mind. I believe I will never see it again in this life.

I remained with the monks for two days, praying and asking the deities to protect us. We spoke of our hopes and our fears. I had no idea what my future would be. I wished only to rejoin Kundun one day. Here at Chothey His Holiness's return was so much hoped for. Before I left, I examined the oldest monks and prescribed some medicinal substances. Doubtless they felt and concealed a certain pride that I had originally been one of them.

Very early in the morning I left for my village. I stopped on the way near the monastery of Yentsa. It must have been about eleven o'clock. There were a

few dwellings around the huge building, that also had
suffered destruction by the Chinese. A herd of about
a dozen yaks was grazing peacefully. Children were
working the soil, all the while repeating *Om Mani Padme
Hum*. I approached an adult who was called Dhondup
and we exchanged a few words. He interrupted his
hard labor for a few minutes to go with me as far as
the sanctuary, that opened onto a flowering garden.
A lama who had been a *gueshe*, a doctor of Buddhist
philosophy, at Tashilhunpo came to meet me. Guiding
me through the prayer room and some other rooms, all
richly decorated as in the past, he showed me statues
and effigies representing the Buddha and other divinities. They were magnificent. Butter lamps were
burning before a row of silver offertory bowls. I asked
him how they had been able to preserve all that.

'It is a long story,' he answered, and he took my arm
as we went into the garden, where he served me a bowl
of tea. Two nuns and about fifteen novices sat down
near us. They smiled at me with infinite grace. The
oldest gave me the long account of the events that had
shaken the area around the monastery. At the time of
the Cultural Revolution she had been charged with the
destruction of all the sacred works of Yentsa. Unable to
do anything but submit, she took part in numerous
indoctrination sessions, where she pretended zealous-
ness. Reassured, the Red Guards never noticed the
strange activities that went on in this monastery. Higher
up on the nearby hill there was a small forgotten sanctuary where an old monk still lived. Whenever she
could, the nun would climb up there, one time with a
statue of Buddha, another with an effigy of one of the
deities, then with *thangkas*, or sacred texts rolled up in

old rags. Time would prove to be the best ally of this courageous nun.

On the fifteenth and the twenty-fifth day of every month she went to pray and recite texts with families in the area. One afternoon when she was returning to the monastery she heard the rumble of a drum and fear seized her. The Red Guards had trained Tibetan children to destroy our ancestral traditions and the drum usually announced one of their maneuvers. The nun hurried her step and reached the little sanctuary before the children arrived. She asked the old monk to invoke the protecting deities, then she went down the hill to meet about thirty children who were out of control. With all the firmness she could muster, she asked them what they were doing there.

'We've come to destroy this hellish place.'

Many of the children looked gleeful at the prospect. The beating of the drum grew louder.

'There's nothing for you here,' said the nun. 'I've personally been put in charge of the destruction of the objects. Nothing is left, no statues, no texts. Go away! I've more important things to do than listen to you.'

Convinced by this, the children left and did not come back. I learned that the inhabitants of the area were all supportive of the nuns and that not one of them had ever denounced them. Dhondup said he had had serious difficulties with the Chinese. His son had been arrested in 1966 (the year horse-fire). He himself had been beaten for lighting butter lamps in his house. In spite of the continuous surveillance, Dhondup defied the prohibition and placed a butter lamp inside a Thermos bottle. Unfortunately, the Chinese noticed it and beat him again. To escape the vigilance of his tormentors, Dhondup would climb the hill just before daybreak every morning to light the butter lamps of the monastery. When I returned to Yititok some time later, I made enquiries and found the trail of Dhondup's son. He had been imprisoned at Drapchi but was still alive and I immediately sent him a message.

I remained another two days at the monastery, sharing prayers with the *gueshe* of Tashilhunpo, the nuns and Dhondup. When I left them, I set out in the direction of the village where I had been born. There was still a vast plain and a mountain pass to cross.

I skirted the river whose sinuous course would lead almost to the foot of the hill by my house, the place of all the secrets of my childhood. Way above the snowy peaks I could see vultures turning in a slow looping flight. After a while I turned away from the river, advancing obliquely toward the cliff. A confused thought came back to me, the hoot of the owl I thought I heard in the forest a few days earlier. Perhaps it was only a dream, not necessarily a bad omen. But a rush of dreadful vivid images came to me: the destruction of Chothey, the monks running in all directions to escape the Red Guards, throats slashed, blood flowing, women raped. It was said that on the eve of Communist China's invasion of our country, the mountains, the hills, the rivers gave out strange moans, like distant cannon fire. They said it was the battle that the deities and demons, the protectors of the Dharma, were unleashing against their enemies. The battle raged, like a precursor of the drama that was to envelop us. In Lhasa and its surroundings, just before 10 March, 1959, crows were seen to alight on the ground without making a sound, then point their beaks down and fly off. These things were generally considered bad omens. A few days later the soldiers of our army were massacred.

But here, as far as you could tell, it was peaceful. I thought only about my family. *Mola* must be a very old woman. I smiled at the memory of the stories about Aku Tempa that *Pala* would tell in the evenings by the fire. As I climbed the hill to the house, I heard dogs howling. The owl in my dream, these dogs in this early morning hour – were they signs of bad news to come? My eyes settled on the house where I had been born. My heart was beating hard, so hard . . . The door opened and there stood one of my half-brothers. He stared at me for a second, prostrated himself three times, murmuring: '*Lhamenpa! Lhamenpa!*'

Tears flooded our eyes. A minute later I was in the main room with my family around me, at least what remained of them. The shock was brutal. I learned of *Mola*'s death, and the death of my uncles. I remained with my family for a week. Every day I climbed the hill and stayed for hours praying to Tara, reciting *Mola*'s favorite prayer. I built a miniature temple and planted a prayer flag. One evening when there was a violent storm, the mountain was shaken by an earthquake. A light tremor ran through the house. When calm was restored, a double rainbow appeared in the grey-black sky. I went outside and walked some way up the hill. The rain was falling again and I was soaked. The cold, the darkness, the colors of the rainbow, the rain. I felt ill and fatigued. I closed my eyes and floated in semi-consciousness. *Amala* and *Mola* were smiling at me. I was carried along by waves of emotion that rolled and pitched. *Pala* also had drawn near to me, he took my hand and led me on a path of light. When I came back to myself, I was numb with cold. I saw an eagle take flight. Death was lurking around me. I knew that the least trace of bad karma could follow me, wherever I might be.

'Think about that, Tenzin Choedrak!' I heard myself say aloud.

The conditions of life change from one moment to the next and we suddenly realize that nothing has been accomplished. I must more fully direct what still remained of my life toward the true practice of the Dharma. That was the message from my dear ones. I promised to devote myself to it from that instant without waiting for tomorrow, for death could strike that very evening.

The next day I returned to Lhasa. It took me thirty-six hours of walking. Scarcely had I returned to Yititok, however, than they transferred me to Drapchi. Again! Dr Li had just time to explain to me that it was because of that Chinese who had recently consulted me as a patient and then accused me of conspiring with the 'renegade' Dalai Lama.

16

Twenty-one Years Later

After the death of Mao, China showed a few signs
of interest in opening dialogue. In 1977 Beijing acknowledged regret for certain excesses of the Cultural Revolution. At the time, Ngapo Nouang Jigme, the Tibetan
who had negotiated the 'Seventeen Point Accord' in
1951, which was signed with a counterfeit seal,
had become one of the most important officials of the
Communist regime in Tibet. In a speech he made, he
said he wished for the return of His Holiness and all
the Tibetan refugees. But how could such a person be
believed? A year later, 1978, the local authorities in
Lhasa took a remarkable step: they freed thirty-four
prisoners, who were presented as the 'last great rebel
leaders'. All of this was done with the usual propa-
gandistic fanfare.

Yeche Dordje, a Tibetan doctor from Potangmo, had
approached the Chinese authorities innumerable times
with a request to meet me in Drapchi and he finally
ontained approval. He and two colleagues, Degue
Tsenam and Tsultrim Tensin, had been searching the
country for several years for texts that would allow
them once again to make the precious pills that were no

longer available in Tibet. When we met I told him to go to Ganden and ask on my behalf for Sonam Rinetzine, who I thought would be of help to him. Yeche Dordje finally recovered a copy of the treatise and he met me again, thanks to Pema Choedrak, one of the Tibetan officials of Drapchi. He told me Degue Tsenam had also brought a treatise back from Kham but that neither of them had been able to understand it.

'*Lhamenpa*, you are today the only doctor in Tibet who can make *rine-chen rilbou*. We must put everythng into action to preserve this tradition. Please come with me to Potangmo.'

'I can't go with you and, in the immediate future, that would not accomplish anything,' I said to him. 'On the other hand, you can receive my teachings here.'

Yeche Dordje was authorized to remain in Lhasa and to come to Drapchi every day. It took more than a month to give him a summary of the text, enough for him to return to Potangmo and assemble the ingredients necessary for the fabrication of the pills. A few weeks later I received a visit from Tseguiel Lek. He was the official of Tibetan medicine at Potangmo, of course under the direct control of the Chinese.

'We need you now,' he said to me. 'Don't be afraid. I assume all responsibility for whatever might happen during your stay with us. But before we leave I must confess something to you, *Lhamenpa*. When they spoke to me about you, I pictured an old man.' And he laughed loudly, like Kundun.

'I'm fifty-six years old,' I told him, 'of which I've spent nineteen years in prison.'

Tseguiel Lek did everything to make my journey as smooth as possible. When I arrived at Potangmo I was received with much deference, including by the Chinese doctors who directed the hospital. They took me to Dramtchou, a pleasant place in the middle of meadows crossed by a river. Eighteen prisoners were living and working there under the surveillance of medical students, most of them originally from the region of Kham, notably from Gergue. The dwelling was large and agreeable in comparison with everything that I had known.

The officials of the center had prepared for my arrival. I could examine the ingredients, of which there were about a hundred. I remarked only on the gold, which was not of pure quality. The metal had certainly been confiscated from Tibetans, melted down into balls that were stamped to distinguish it from the other grades of gold that were in the form of ingots or raw extracts. I raised the question with Tseguiel Lek. After three days, I had the response I wanted. They agreed to my request: the gold would come directly from the mines.

It took us four months to obtain about twenty kilos of precious pills. Even though they respected my work, it was not always easy to cohabit with some of the Chinese functionaries and Tibetans. Ordinarily a lama of high rank purifies the mercury and the other metals. Because I was not a high-ranking lama, I was derided. But I refused to let myself be caught up in their stupid game and went about my work. The conditions were not ideal and it required considerable energy from everyone involved. It did not help that the guards regularly insisted on quenching their own and everybody else's thirst with glasses of *chang*. But I believe that the deities and the guardians of the Dharma were with me. The medicines were ready by the time of the harvests, which proved to be excellent, much better even than in preceding years. A Tibetan woman came to inform me of it. I answered with a knowing smile:

'The texts say that to obtain a good harvest, you must first purify some mercury. It's even better if you also prepare other metals.'

The woman left reassured and henceforth they thought of me as a sage and a fine interpreter of supernatural things.

A three- or four-hour walk from Dramtchou were other prisons: Tchamdo, Nandak, Traloung, Guchang, and Zongnak, some of which had the reputation of being terribly harsh. Although my sentence had ended more than two years ago, I was still living under the control of the Chinese prison authorities. No-one had yet mentioned my release and I no longer much believed in it. I had to go regularly to the Zongnak camp, the furthest one from Dramtchou. I would leave very early in the morning and arrive around noon. Tseguiel Lek had suggested that I prepare medicines for the prisoners and the personnel of the camp. We could not prescribe the precious pills for them because the high-ranking officers would certainly have diverted them for themselves and their families. So we made a substance that also contained mercury, but in lesser amounts. On each of my visits I saw patients and gave them these substances that afforded them a little relief.

A river ran around Zongnak. Water from a makeshift pipe that crossed the camp permitted the soldiers and camp personnel to wash their clothes. This dirty water, which ran down into a ditch, is what the prisoners drank. Those who consumed it invariably fell ill. One day a Tibetan woman closed off the ditch with dirt, but the Chinese noticed and imposed a *thamzing* session on her. The ditch was reopened, the prisoners continued to be infected. When they complained to the camp doctor, they were told they were simply claiming to be sick to get out of working.

Attempts at escape were rare. When it happened, the men were humiliated, tortured, and led to the edge of the nearby cliff where they were killed with a bullet in the neck and three more in the heart. The bodies were thrown into the river. As soon as spring arrived, the camp was filled with a nauseating odor. Shreds of flesh and bone often floated in the pipeline. In the course of one of my visits to Nandak I learned that eighteen prisoners had attempted to escape. A hole about ten meters wide was dug and the prisoners were lined up at the edge and machine-gunned. The other prisoners were then assembled and warned that death awaited anyone who attempted to escape from the camp. Such stories abounded. There was one about an old man who boasted of having eaten a montain goat. Someone overheard him telling this and misunderstood the Tibetan word for mountain goat, which is an abbreviation of the word for 'Chinese'. Suspected of having eaten a soldier, he remained incarcerated for three long years. A guard was talking to him one day and out of curiosity asked him:

'But what did you do with the clothes?'

'Have you ever seen a mountain goat wearing clothes?' asked the good man, flabbergasted. He was fortunate enough to be released. Many others died innocent.

The house where we stayed at Dramtchou had been built with the stones from a monastery. The mantras were still visible in the stones. The floor was tiled with a picture of the Buddha and a mandala. It was more and more common in Tibet to see public places, notably toilets for tourists or for the army, built with what remained of the sanctuaries or the sacred mural paintings.

Returning to Dramtchou from the Zongnak camp late one afternoon, I met a little boy. He could not have been more than ten years old. I sat down next to him for a few minutes.

'Tell me, when will we be free? When will the Chinese leave?'

His questions immediately aroused my mistrust. I turned the question back to him.

'Why are you questioning me like that? Why ask me that?'

'*Pala* died in a camp and since then *Amala* is beaten every day by the villagers.'

'What do they have against her?'

'For being the wife of a reactionary,' he sobbed.

Then he told me his mother had run away and that she wanted to kill herself. She had already thrown her youngest child into the river.

'I'm the oldest and she's looking for me everywhere.'

I learned later that the Tibetan woman finally did commit suicide. I entrusted the boy to the care of one of my patients, who advised me to remain on my guard because of the numerous spies in the area.

When I was still at Drapchi, before leaving for Potangmo, I had proposed to the Chinese authorities that they open a branch of Men-Tsee-Khang to care for the prisoners and the outside patients who wanted to meet me. When I came back to Drapchi in Lhasa, I found that my request had been granted. I felt a profound satisfaction but was aware of the difficulty of the task that awaited me. Many medicinal substances were lacking. I left with a group of prisoners, including Seupa, Domkou, Tseten Namguiel, Sonam, Pelden, Guelek, and about thirty others, to collect plants in the immediate area. Trucks were waiting for us at the foot of the mountain. We returned to Drapchi when they were loaded. As we passed through villages I noticed that Tibetans were selling medicinal plants for small sums in shops run by Chinese. The good quality herbs were sent to China, the others sold retail to the Tibetans. When I needed substances not available in Nepal, India, or China, I had to send a letter to the prison director, who then authorized me to buy them in the Chinese shops of Lhasa.

The Chinese pursued the massive felling of trees with the use of dynamite in the area around Lhasa. You could see places here and there where the forest had entirely disappeared, and with it the plants, the flowers, all the flora and fauna of which we Tibetans were so respectful. The trees were very old and often enormous, and it was impossible to uproot them by hand. The prisoners dug around the roots and the guards placed the sticks of explosives. The tree seemed to shudder an instant and then fell. The trunk, stripped of its banches, was sent thundering down the slope. They were sent to the sawmill; the best cuts went to China, the others were sold and used mainly for firewood.

During these stays on the mountain we were usually lodged in a tent, although sometimes we went down into the valley and were received by the local people. I always took advantage of this to meet patients. I had to limit myself to examining them and prescribing medicines that they would then have to procure on their own. Everywhere I encountered misery. You could see the fear in people's eyes. Everyone told me about the terrible atrocities that the Chinese continued to commit. It would happen that families would bring *thankgas*, effigies of divinities, a small statue of the Buddha, out of hiding just long enough to invoke the deities. I prayed with them and as soon as we finished, the sacred objects were put back in their hiding places. I also met nomads, some of whom pastured their yaks on the immensity of the high plateaus. Tents outlined their camps. The first one was often used for storing milk, butter, and dried meat. All these foodstuffs were regularly collected by the Chinese, who left only a meager part to the nomads.

At the time I might have thought of trying to escape. I did not do it because leaving to go to India and rejoin the Dalai Lama also meant abandoning my compatriots and causing them to lose the slight possibility that remained to them of receiving care. Besides, if I reached the mountain, my escape would put the other prisoners in danger of retribution. There were certainly attempts at escape and some succeeded. People could not put themselves at too much risk in coming to the aid of prisoners; danger was everywhere, even in the person of your brother or your neighbor.

In 1979 (the year sheep-earth) I learned that the United States had officially recognized China. That year the Panchen Lama reappeared in Lhasa after many years of imprisonment. Was this a sign of hope? We knew that the Dalai Lama continued to travel the world to inform about Tibet's desperate situation. His Holiness had also asked Beijing to allow the exiles who wished to see their families again to return to Tibet. One day I learned that a Tibetan delegation led by Lobsang Samden, one of the Dalai Lama's brothers, had left Delhi for Tibet. It was 2 August, 1979. The delegation remained in Tibet for four months. When they arrived in the capital, on 1 October, tens of thousands of people were assembled around Norbulingka, the former summer residence of the Dalai Lama, which had been transformed into an immense 'people's park'. This was a Chinese holiday. I was free that day and would be able to go into Norbulingka. I was accompanied by Seupa, Phunetsok, Sonam, Pelden, and Doungtouk, who was a relative of the regent Reting Rinpoche, who had directed the administration of the country when the Dalai Lama was still a minor. We had brought along a little *chang* and some *tsampa*. The closer we came to Norbulingka, the denser the crowd. Shouts drowned out the voices of His Holiness's representatives. Women wept and some fainted. Men elbowed their way through to protect Lobsang Samden and his companions. We gathered our energy to cross the last few meters that separated us from the delegation. My companions practically carried me along. And then I saw them.

'Lobsang Samden!'

'*Lhamenpa*! *Lhamenpa*! Come quickly!'

I had recognized Lobsang Samden. But something had changed in his profile, it was that now he had a mustache and his hair was full. Twenty years later! My throat knotted. I had difficulty controlling my emotion. Lobsang Samden, Ngari Rinpoche, Thubten Jigme Norbou, Jetsune Pema, *Amala*, and . . . Kundun.

But only Lobsang Samden was there. I presented him with a *kata*.

'How happy I am to see you, *Lhamenpa*. To know you are in Lhasa, alive. *Amala*, Kundun, everyone will be so happy at this news, doubtless the best of our journey, for all the rest is desolation. What horrors! What shame!'

My emotion made it impossible for me to speak, and then the immense crowd was shouting: 'Long live a free Tibet! Tibet for the Tibetans! Long live the Dalai Lama! Long life to Kundun!'

Surveying the vast crowd of Tibetans who had come to draw near to His Holiness's brother, one of the Chinese officials who was accompanying and watching the delegation said, 'A single day has been enough to wipe out twenty years of effort.' While we exchanged a few words, my group protected the delegation by pushing back as best we could this human wave, at once so terrifying and beautiful, full of the hopes of an entire population.

We met a little later away from observation, and Lobsang Samden talked to me about the life of Tibetan refugees, about the government in exile, the travels of His Holiness, the more and more favorable reverberation of our cause in public opinion.

'And you, *Lhamenpa*? How have you survived?'

I did not answer this question. We were being observed by some Chinese but the Tibetan informers, seated next to us, were even more dangerous. I lied to Lobsang Samden.

'Everything is fine. Since the motherland began the renewal of Tibet, there have been many changes. The Tibetans are now less ignorant and we have an agreeable life.'

Of all of us, Phunetsok seemed the most moved. Suddenly he grabbed the hand of the Dalai Lama's brother and began to tell him what had really happened in Tibet since the departure of Kundun and his entourage. Someone photographed the scene. Lobsang Samden talked to me for a long while about *Amala*. She was asking for me in Dharamsala.

'It's not possible. I have no reason to leave Tibet. I am useful to my compatriots. But if you really wish me to come to India you must speak to the Chinese authorities who give me my orders.'

The Dalai Lama's brother looked straight into my eyes, shrugged his shoulders, a gesture of powerlessness. Our conversation revealed nothing of the truth. Lobsang Samden murmured a few words to me, while Seupa and Phunetsok distracted the attention of the informers. Another meeting was arranged. At nightfall I went to the hotel where the delegation was staying. There were many Chinese but the guards did not intrude. I could finally speak with Lobsang Samden without a witness and I told him everything that I had seen and lived.

The delegation departed from Lhasa and left behind it an immense wave of hope and expectation. The Tibetans spoke of Kundun's return, the end of repression. Even in the prisons and the camps, the prisoners could not hide their joy. But alas, nothing really changed for them. The Chinese authorities let a few days go by, then gathered the highest officials of the Autonomous Region, and also called the Tibetans who were in league with them and some of the prisoners. I was also invited to this assembly as the representative of the Tibetan medical community.

The speeches were long-winded. Finally we learned that Beijing intended to further develop Tibet, and that it expected from us suggestions, ideas and critiques, in order that we might all prepare a better future for the Tibetan people. There were Chinese doctors at the conference. They announced the construction of a traditional Western hospital which I was able to see the next day. The building was already well under way. It was then that the officials informed me of their intention to make me the head of the center for Tibetan medicine. Aware that during the Cultural Revolution the medical treatises had been burned, they proposed that I begin the editing of a work that would be useful for future generations.

In my heart, the proposal did not displease me, because I would be preserving our ancestral traditions. It was necessary at all costs to reassemble the ancient texts that might have been saved. I warned the officials who were present about the difficulties of editing such a work. I also made the point of the imperative necessity to collect medicinal substances before opening the center, because they were more and more scarce and Men-Tsee-Khang could no longer respond to all the demands. I remembered that the Red Guards had thrown hundreds of kilos of medicinal powders into cesspits and that such a thing should never happen again. I also demanded paper and support. I obtained everything. My salary of thirty yuan was no longer sufficient, it was raised to sixty yuan. Eighty Tibetans came to help me in the preparation of the work. Thus, in a few weeks, I was able to reassemble some ancient treatises.

I also organized the collection of the plants. Teams

composed only of prisoners and led by young doctors left regularly for different sites in the region. At the foot of Men-Tsee-Khang grew a sort of radish, the roots of which we used. I took some to mix with other substances and had it replanted near Drapchi. Later, I discovered that this plant grew in abundance in the Spiti, on the border of India and Tibet.

We lacked space at Drapchi, so the local Chinese authorities authorized me to use as storage space the empty cells of the monastery of Sera, whose facade was being reconstructed. I could work on site to supervise the drying and transformation stages, always on condition that I return every evening to Drapchi, except for special authorization. I would always be a pawn in the hands of the Chinese! Normally I would have been released in 1976 (the year dragon-fire). Three years later, I was still considered a prisoner, even if I was now able to treat patients, both Chinese and Tibetans.

Going regularly to and from Drapchi, I had gotten into the habit of walking around the temple. One day I heard two girls talking about changes that had occurred here.

'All our monasteries are in ruins,' one of them exclaimed. 'The Chinese re-do the facades to lure the Tibetans and the tourists. But the interiors are so miserable!'

The situation was identical to that of Sera, which was partly rebuilt for tourism. But inside, all the statues, the effigies, and the sacred objects had disappeared. To hear these young girls talk of our culture filled my heart with confidence. In twenty-nine years of occupation, the Chinese had not succeeded in breaking us.

Since I could not leave the immediate area of Lhasa

without special permission, I managed to find sub-stances imported from India, Nepal, and China in a shop near Drapchi whose owners were my patients. The only customer of this supplier was Men-Tsee-Khang. I knew which ingredients they had in stock. I had also gotten into the habit of making a list of the powders I needed and having it signed by the director of Drapchi, an angry Chinese who one day accused me of running a business. From then on, he refused to give his signature. Fortunately, the people of the shop were very under-standing and continued to make deliveries to me, no longer at Drapchi but at Sera.

In the past, the monastery of Sera had been a humming city. Now, it was in ruins and for the most part was abandoned. A few monks loafed about, waiting for possible tourists. We could therefore easily store the plants here, but we first had to clean the empty cells and repair the gutted roofs. Because we lacked tools, we had to prepare the powders by crushing them with large rocks on the stone benches in what had been the monastery garden. Some prisoners from Drapchi helped me and returned with me every evening to the camp.

In 1980 (the year monkey-iron) a new delegation urged on by the Dalai Lama and led by his younger sister, Jetsune Pema, arrived in Lhasa. An earlier mission of inquiry composed of young people had been expelled under the pretext that they were stirring rebellion. During the one hundrd and twenty-five days that the long journey lasted, from 1 June to 3 October, the group traveled thirteen thousand kilometers. Every-where that Jetsune Pema and her friends went, people spoke of the 'errors' committed by the Gang of Four, but they still dared to claim that now everything was going very well in the Tibet they were visiting. Contrary to Beijing's affirmations, the major part of our cultural and religious patrimony had been destroyed between 1956 and 1961, and not during the famous Cultural Revolution (1966–1976). Of a total of more than six thousand monasteries and convents, there remained only eight by 1976 (the year dragon-fire).

When Jetsune Pema's presence was announced in the capital, a crowd of several thousand people assembled again at Norbulingka where she gave a remarkable speech, mentioning the health of His Holiness and the efforts of the Tibetans in exile who, like us, were pursuing two principal objectives: the return of Kundun and the liberation of Tibet. Emotions were intense and the Chinese were on the alert. When at four o'clock in the morning I met Jetsune Pema at her hotel, we were both very moved. From the window of her room she could see the Potala, still so majestic. In a room on the next to the top floor, a little light twinkled.

'Apart from a caretaker, no-one lives there any more,' I confided to her with regret.

She spoke to me a bit about the trip, of what she had been able to ascertain, and told me that it pained her greatly to see the Tibetans reduced to the condition of quasi-slaves. In the cities, most of them were forced to beg, the schools were closed. Famine persisted in the country. Jetsune Pema discovered a city quite different from the one she had known. It had been almost entirely destroyed and buildings in the Chinese style replaced the old ones. She experienced a profound sadness when she went to Chang-Sep-Char. The family dwelling had been transformed into an inn for Chinese officers. The grillwork was filled in and the windows painted blue. The city's sewers overflowed and there was no longer any flushing of water. There were light fixtures and light bulbs, but no electricity because the current was available only in the areas where the Chinese lived. She was surprised that the people of Lhasa always walked with their heads down. I explained to her that during the Cultural Revolution they were denied the right to raise their eyes, and they had kept the habit ever since. They still lived in perpetual fear of reprisals. The investigative mission found that all the radio programs were broadcast in Chinese. In the evening indoctrination sessions were imposed on the population, veritable brainwashings which began at sundown and often went on until the early morning.

Jetsune Pema talked to me about *Amala*'s fragile health and said that she suffered from hypertension. She told me that a request had been made to the Chinese authorities to allow me to go to India for a few months to visit the Dalai Lama's mother.

The request was granted and I had permission to leave for three months. I immediately informed Jetsune Pema and gave her an enormous sack containing very old sacred texts, notably medical treatises, for safekeeping. I knew that the Chinese would never let me take them away and that I would be searched, whereas the delegation could take them in their baggage without too much risk. Just before my departure from Lhasa in October 1980 Pema Choedrak, a very influential Tibetan official in the capital, came to see me.

'I know,' he said, 'that you will not come back.'

'Why such a statement?' I asked.

I was terribly mistrustful because this man was not stupid. He knew that in leaving Tibet, I would be rejoining the Dalai Lama and his government in exile.

'Since the end of the Cultural Revolution, many things have changed in Tibet. We need people like you. We still intend to award you an important post at the center for Tibetan medicine. Why go to India?'

'I have nothing to say to you about it,' I answered him. 'On the other hand, if you really want to help me, lend me a little money. I cannot borrow in India, it would be shameful for the motherland.'

'How much do you need?'

'I only earn sixty yuan a month and I can't finance such a trip. I would need a thousand yuan, which I will pay back on my return.'

Pema Choedrak finally agreed to lend me this amount, convinced that he would never be reimbursed.

At the moment that I entered Jokhang to pray to the deities, I suddenly became aware of how much the Chinese had undermined our religion. With the exception of a few statues and some sacred texts, everything that had to do closely or remotely with Buddhism had been destroyed. Without these objects to venerate, most Tibetans felt lost. Some had hidden them away, at the risk of their lives.

After twenty-one years of imprisonment, these three months of leave were a sign. I thought that now my life would improve. 'The Karma engenders everything,' said the Buddha. The fact of having suffered so much allowed me to draw nearer to other human beings, sensitized me, perhaps more than others, to the terrible situation of Tibet. I was always extremely cautious because no-one knew what might yet happen. I could not forget all those years that I saw so many of my compatriots succumb under the torture of our Chinese jailers. Even if I now felt serene, I could not say that I was happy. My people continued to suffer and these sufferings have not ceased since the Communist occupation in 1949. Every day still, women, sometimes very old, and children cross the Himalayan chain to find refuge and protection with His Holiness the Dalai Lama. My analysis would perhaps be otherwise if I learned that the Tibetans now enjoy a certain freedom. Unfortunately, that is far from true.

Before leaving the city, I visited the principal sanctuaries for a last time and met some of my family. I told them that once I was in Dharamsala, I would never write to them, but they should not be concerned. I was fifty-eight years old, and I already felt so old! For the rest of my life, I wanted to be with the Yapchi family, do my best to serve the Dalai Lama and his government, and, if possible, help my compatriots to overcome their suffering.

The morning of my departure, a rainbow enveloped the Potala, the former residence of Kundun. An intense emotion gripped me. I was leaving my country, perhaps not to see it again in this life. It was four o'clock when I crossed the Kyitchou river. At eight o'clock, I stopped to drink some tea and eat a little *tsampa*. At the moment of crossing the first pass, I turned around a last time. The Potala shone under a thousand fires of the sun. All

along the road I recited a personal appeal to the deities
of the Dharma:

> *Help us regain our freedom soon,*
> *Help us recover our independence,*
> *Allow us to return,*
> *Long life to Kundun!*

17

Again With Kundun

At the end of October 1980 (the year monkey-iron) I left
Lhasa. I felt happy and, at the same time, I was haunted
by the thought that my compatriots would continue
to endure atrocities while I was walking to freedom.
Staying with a maternal aunt, I spent several weeks at
Kathmandu, visiting the sacred places of Buddhism. In
the morning I walked around the sites, while in the
afternoon I saw patients. I reached New Delhi by plane
and traveled up to Dharamsala, where I arrived in the
early morning hours.

Four o'clock, the first movements of the dawn:
rustling of robes, flickering light of butter lamps, plumes
of incense, soft steps, old hands playing over a worn
mala. The day was breaking. Men and women were bent
over, walking with little steps, along the *lingkor*, the path
that runs around the temple and the residence of His
Holiness. I followed the same path, once, twice, three
times. Like them I took a few steps, knelt, rose, took a
few more steps. On the small open space bordered with
trees facing the temple of Tsouklagkhang, there were
other shadowy figures bent in prayer. All my thoughts
were turned to the Dalai Lama, whom I would see again

either today or the next day. With the murmured prayers, the pain left my body and I felt strangely light. I lost myself in the prayer flags that fluttered in the wind. I stopped before the *mani* stones to meditate and offer homage to our dead.

The buildings had been hastily constructed with roofs of cardboard, metal plates, sometimes wood. It was simple but frequently miserable, as if the Tibetan refugees lived there only in the expectation of leaving, in the unique hope of a return already unconsciously programmed. Some had been living in Dharamsala for twenty years, since the installation of the Dalai Lama and his government in exile. I noted the same fervor in my compatriots. As I walked about, I noticed in a dwelling an altar lit with little butter lamps that diffused a twinkling brightness on a pot of buttered salted tea or perhaps *toukpa-baktouk*, the traditional soup common in all the regions of our country. In a corner, a woman was preparing *tsampa* or steamed bread. An old man was murmuring *Om Mani Padme Hum* . . . Life here was far from peaceful, but it was always entirely colored with fervor and compassion. At Mc Leod Ganj, the high part of the village, some inscriptions on the walls or the wooden barracks – 'Save Tibet' and 'Tibet is still alive!' – reminded me that most of my brothers and sisters were still living under Chinese occupation. I was especially struck by seeing Western Buddhist monks for the first time. I had noticed some in Nepal a few days earlier, but that had been just a fleeting glimpse. When I saw them in Dharamasala, I knew the Chinese would never vanquish the sons and daughters of the Dharma. The work of the Buddha would continue, thanks also to the wisdom of our sovereign who tirelessly pursued his duty to deliver his precious teachings.

That afternoon Kundun welcomed me warmly. He asked me to tell him of the suffering of our people in the Chinese jails, and also my own. I had to describe my prison experiences several times. Later, even in the street, Tibetans would stop me to ask questions. His Holiness wanted me to bear witness to our exiled compatriots in Dharamsala, so that all might become aware of the drama that had been unfolding in our country since 1949. He proposed that I resume my position as his personal physician. I accepted with such profound, intense joy that tears flooded my eyes. After so many years of suffering and obstacles, life finally seemed to smile on me again.

The Dalai Lama had not changed. He still had that same cosmic laugh and shone with that same energetic spirit. The only difference was that with age, he was now forty-five years old, his abilities were even greater. He did admit to me that his travels throughout the world greatly tired him, but that was nothing compared with what the Tibetan people were enduring. At that time, there was no question of my accompanying him on his trips abroad. Then we spoke of *Amala*'s delicate health.

As tradition willed it, the audience with His Holiness terminated and I then visited Gyalyoum* Chenmo, the honorific title given to the Dalai Lama's mother, who was living at Kashmir Cottage. *Amala* was eighty years old, and I had decided to be prudent in answering the questions that I knew she would ask about conditions in Tibet. *Amala* was aware of the atrocities committed by the Chinese and she knew that the horrors had never stopped. Jetsune Pema must have told her everything. So when I saw her, once the emotion had quieted, she assailed me with a flood of questions, especially concerning my life in the prisons. She had been informed in large part about my fate, but she wanted to hear it from me. *Amala* had been suffering for a long time from hypertension and had had a stroke that paralyzed her whole left side, so that she had to be helped to walk. But, more than her illness, it was the condition of the Tibetan people that made her suffer horribly. Since her departure from Lhasa in 1959, she kept hoping to return to her country and, especially, to end her days in Taktser in the Amdo, although she knew this would never come to pass.

The winter of 1980 was particularly harsh in Dharamsala. There were heavy snowfalls. Despite the difficulty of getting around, I visited the different departments of the central administration, Health, Education, Finance, Religious Affairs, International Relations and Information, and Justice. Family planning would be added in 1988. I was received by the *Kashag* and by the Assembly which held a special session. I learned about the democratic structures put in place by His Holiness the Dalai Lama. We had a government in exile that functioned on the model of many other countries. Our deputies, today numbering forty-six, were elected for five years and they named the seven members of the *Kashag*, who in turn appointed their president. There was only one dark cloud over this picture: the Tibetan government in exile was not recognized by any nation.

It was at this period that I again saw Jetsune Pema, Kundun's younger sister. She was president of the Tibetan Children's Village, which she had been directing since the year dragon-wood (1964), the year of the death of the eldest daughter, Tsering Deulma. Jetsune Pema and her team had just celebrated their twentieth anniversary in the presence of our sovereign. I was impressed by all the work accomplished since our government in exile had been established in 1960 [the year mouse-iron] in Dharamsala. What a long road traveled, so much suffering assuaged, and obstacles overcome! I felt very proud and emotional looking at these children. The joy came from seeing them wreathed in smiles, surrounded by adoptive parents in homes that were continually being built. Yet it was sad to see newcomers arriving every day who were still fleeing the Chinese atrocities.

Frequently I visited *Amala*, who had always expended all her energy in supporting her children, especially Kundun and Jetsune Pema, and helping all the refugees who arrived in Dharamsala, often in a pitiable state both physically and mentally. I also requested another audience with His Holiness, during which I would officially resume my responsibilities. It finally took place with the dignity and simplicity required for such a ceremony. Two young doctors were presented with me and I was to train them so they could succeed me if something happened to me. Kundun received our *katas* and announced our appointments. When the audience ended, I went to the temple of Tsouklagkhang to pray to the deities of medicine. I said this prayer, among others:

> *Let there be no enemies,*
> *Let there be no curses,*
> *Let there be no illness,*

> *May all conflict cease,*
> *May happiness grow in minds and bodies,*
> *May there be riches and strength,*
> *May richness abound in the grains of our land,*
> *May I still live a long time,*
> *And may all my wishes come to pass.*
> *Long life to Kundun!*
> *Long life to the Yapchi family!*

A few weeks later, my rank (the fifth) in the Tibetan hierarchy was restored and the Dalai Lama appointed me, beginning in 1962, to the board of directors of Men-Tsee-Khang, which he was adamant about restoring despite enormous difficulties.

Years later Kundun wanted to entrust to me a very different mission. It would prove to be important.

During this time *Amala*'s health worsened and she died on 12 January, 1981 (the year bird-iron). Gyalyoum Chenmo's death caused deep sadness in our little community and the pain could be read on everyone's face. The population was in a state of shock and prepared for forty-nine days of mourning.

Every morning, I would go to Kundun's residence to take his pulse. A single day did not go by without His Holiness speaking to me about Men-Tsee-Khang, which had occupied a tiny building at Mc Leod Ganj since 1962. He said to me:

'Take it in hand. Like education, like the opera, we must preserve our medicine.'

Financed in the beginning from the Dalai Lama's personal funds and later by donations, Men-Tsee-Khang had gone through numerous internal problems. The doctors wanted to leave. Some had already left for purely financial reasons. One of them had opened a private clinic that occupied a large site and she was making the medicines herself. I could not understand such behavior because we needed every available medical professional to preserve the work of my venerable master, Khenrab Norbu, and his eminent predecessors. 'The old doctors could read the pulse just by touching the patient's shoelaces,' they used to say in Tibet. Things were very different today and I regretted it.

Having completed my assessment of what the institute needed, I went to see Lobsang Samden, who directed it at the time. I asked him if they were making the precious pills and whether the doctors knew how to go about purifying the metals, such as gold and, especially, mercury. He told me that they had at most only eighty different medicines. The situation was serious. Some precious pills, which did not come from Men-Tsee-Khang but from certain doctors, not entirely scrupulous, were available on the market but lacked the essential substances. I mentioned this to the Dalai Lama's administration, who told me that they were quite aware of the problem, but there was no money. I said that we would lose all our patients if a solution could not be found quickly. The situation could not continue.

One morning in the course of a consultation I decided to speak to His Holiness about it. I proposed to him that we make the least complex precious pills and the Dalai Lama agreed to my request. I immediately asked Tsarong Jigme, who was then living in Ladakh, to bring me the basic ingredients. He came to Dharamsala

with a small bottle that he handed me. I laughed, somewhere between amusement and irritation.

'What do you expect me to do with that? One bottle
isn't good for anything.'

'There are so many substances available in Ladakh,
Lhamenpa. You ought to come.'

But I could not because we had already spent a lot of
money to pay for Tsarong Jigme's plane fare.

'All your words are as useless as bubbles, but I don't
doubt that you have done your best,' I told him.

Over a few months a more efficient organization
took form. We were beginning to receive medicinal
plants from Tibet and basic substances from certain
mountainous regions of India. The Dalai Lama gave
me a hundred thousand rupees, about three thousand
pounds, for the construction of a new building, where
the Men-Tsee-Khang of Dharamsala is now located.
Then we needed large quantities of coal to heat
the gold, copper, and silver to transform them into
powders. The preparation of the *tsotru* required about a
hundred ingredients and we received the authorization
to prepare the medicines behind the residence of His
Holiness, on a spot where Kundun regularly made ritual
fires.

Between the second and sixth month of 1982 (the year
dog-water), we worked hard under the encouraging
and protecting gaze of our spiritual guide. We obtained
three million *rin-chen tsotro dachel* pills, that we sold for
five rupees apiece. Sometimes, the silence at the end of
the day would be broken by the sound of His Holiness
laughing. Tsarong Jigme and I lived in a small house
situated near our work site, because we needed to keep
an eye on the fire and especially the purification process

of the metals. Now that we were in possession of fifteen million rupees, we could think about the next step. The day arrived when we were able to produce sufficient quantities of our most highly reputed medicines, *rin-chen drangdjor rilnak chenmo* and *rin-chen ratna sampel*. It was a great victory for us.

At this time, I became aware that we were wasting much of the basic materials. Certain substances could not be ground fine enough by hand to be usable. We absolutely had to have grinding machines. I explained this to His Holiness and told him that the Chinese had installed this type of machine at Men-Tsee-Khang in Lhasa. The opinion of the Dalai Lama's advisors was also sought, for Dharamsala is one of the dampest regions of India and nothing guaranteed the success of our project. Finally Kundun agreed to my proposal and I said to the sceptics, of whom there were many:

'The world makes progress every day. You can see it here, in India. Should we continue to remain rooted in the past when we have the possibility of moving forward? With the old methods that you advocate, we would need several hundred people for months and there are only fifteen of us.'

I found the types of machines that we needed in Bombay. Their arrival in Dharamsala caused a stir. Even the students of Men-Tsee-Khang reacted. 'These look like tanks. What a waste to have spent so much money . . .'

I was in the refugee camps in the south of India when word of the objections to the machines reached me and I was a little discouraged by it. That evening I meditated and prayed to the deities to help me. A few weeks later, his private secretary informed me that His Holiness

283

wanted to pay a visit and see the machines. I put them into operation and my team produced nearly two thousand kilos of incense. Kundun was very attracted by anything technical. When he saw the machines grinding, he burst out laughing and congratulated all of us. His Holiness the Dalai Lama, Tenzin Namguiel and I posed for posterity in front of our famous machines.

Now we had to create a medical school. There was none in Dharamsala. In the beginning we had five students. Confronted with the difficulties of the task, two of them left; but other candidates applied and there were soon ten students. I had a tent set up where the kitchen is now located, and we took our meals there together; to cook we used kerosene that blackened the walls. But it was difficult to house the students. Later, on a trip to Italy, Namguielo Lhamo, the wife of Lobsang Samden, and I obtained sponsorship for our school. It was thanks to these gifts that the large building of the present Men-Tsee-Khang was built at a cost of more than ten million rupees. The kitchen was financed by the sale of precious pills. At this time I was staying at the Hotel Kokonor in Dharamsala. Once, during our absence, a pack of monkeys came down, wreaking havoc in the room and making off with everything they could find, such as clothing and soap.

In 1984 (the year mouse-wood) five dispensaries of Tibetan medicine were opened, one in Mundgod, two in Bylakouppe, and two others in Dharamsala. To meet the needs of the numerous patients, we had to expand our plant-collection activity. I will necessarily be a little vague about this so as not to endanger the families and the Tibetan military who were sent into certain regions on the border of Tibet, on the Indian side, to help me collect the plants that we needed. These men, commanded by an Indian officer, carried out remarkable and difficult work. I myself once even had to take a helicopter, which I nicknamed the 'squalling airplane'. The place was so steep that I had to use a walking stick to climb the slope. Some of us had mountain sickness. Everywhere we went the second in command, who was leading the group, signaled our position by radio. We were able to collect eighty sacks of extremely pure medicinal plants.

Once the medicines were prepared, we decided to distribute them free to the Tibetan refugees and the Indian patients who were beginning to come to consult us. In New Delhi we had installed a medical center in the Tibet House and we were lodged twenty minutes from there in a house that had been very kindly put at our disposal. It was also at this time that the Indian minister of health, a woman, advised us to open a center for traditional Tibetan medicine.

'How do you expect us to do that?' I asked her. 'We have no land.'

A few days later, we met with officials of the Indian capital. They advised us first to rent a house, which we occupied two years before buying it. A little later I addressed a meeting of Tibetan doctors and I told them that we desperately needed qualified personnel for the dispensaries.

I was very surprised at how the qualities needed for helping others were sometimes diverted to personal enrichment. I could have followed this path, had I chosen to, but I did not do so, because the Tibetan people needed competent professionals. Centers opened at

Kollegal, Bangalorem with the help of Tenpa Tsering, then in Nepal, in Sikkim, and in Ladakh. There are today about forty of these clinics. For all these places we acquired buildings financed by the funds of Men-Tsee-Khang, which was now receiving aid from more and more benefactors, and always from His Holiness the Dalai Lama. The donors were American, Japanese, English, French. My salary was close to three hundred rupees a month [about ten dollars].

In Dharamsala at around six o'clock in the morning I would go twice a week, on Monday and Thursday, to the residence of His Holiness the Dalai Lama. I would take his pulse. I must say that our sovereign was very robust and suffered from no serious illness. Since he became the spiritual and temporal leader of Tibet at the age of sixteen, he had always worked very hard. Sometimes on his trips he was so busy that he did not even have time to eat. These were the occasions when I noticed certain fluctuations in his condition, but it was never very serious. I sometimes had to ask him not to consume so much sweet tea or fatty food, like peanut butter. Today, the Dalai Lama asks for traditional as often as for Western medicine. He regularly has check-ups. Most of the time, the two diagnoses are in agreement, but he says he prefers to take Tibetan medicines.

In 1985 (the year cattle-wood) His Holiness asked me to participate in a series of conferences in the West. Invited by great masters, such as Dagpo Rinpoche in France or Sogyal Rinpoche in Great Britain, I took a flight from New Delhi. I discovered Europe, i.e. Italy, Germany, and Switzerland with its many Tibetan refugees, before going to Australia and the United States at the invitation of some others. I participated in numerous conferences and debates with Western doctors. I remember especially the day at Harvard when, before thirty-seven Western medical specialists, I had to take the pulse of several patients. I was uneasy but everything went very well. My diagnoses proved to be exact and precise. I then spoke at length about the *loung*, the humor that governs the functions of exchanges, such as respiration, expectoration, muscular activity, speech, menstruation, urination, and matters related to the nervous system. In London, I participated in a discussion in a center specializing in the treatment of cancer.

I was fatigued and sometimes irritated by the succession of meetings, each more important than the last one. I knew also that some of these people were testing the reliability of our medicine. At the time, we had undertaken research into cancer, AIDS, obesity, asthma, diabetes, and other serious illnesses, including cardiac problems that I discovered in many of the patients on my different trips. At the beginning of the exile, the Tibetan refugees were decimated by tuberculosis, an illness that was almost unknown in Tibet.

With our teams scouring the bordering regions and countries in search of medicinal plants, I made an observation. In 1727 Tenzin Phunestok, one of the most famous specialists of the Tibetan pharmacopoeia, compiled the list of some 2,294 medicinal substances, besides commenting on and testing 312. Today we use hardly 1,500 substances and 200 species of plants. These are our capital, the treasure from which we prepare the most indispensable medicines.

There is no question of taking short cuts in any of the

preparations, under the pretext that we have trouble locating the necessary ingredients. I truly believe the Dalai Lama would not accept it, because he has proven to be more and more demanding in everything that concerns Men-Tsee-Khang.

As the months went by, I had to juggle the training of young Tibetan doctors with my conferences throughout the world. It was difficult, all the more so because Men-Tsee-Khang's success was growing. In Dharamsala, we received visits from foreign doctors. In 1986 (the year tiger-fire) I learned of the tragedy that struck the inhabitants of Chernobyl on 26 April of that year. Three years later, in 1989, I had the opportunity to go to the Soviet Union to visit the sites contaminated by the catastrophe. The Ukrainian population was suffering terribly. A meeting had been organized with other doctors. In the course of this meeting, I made reference to our medical texts which, in the eleventh century, touched on questions of contamination linked to the progress of humanity and to chemical experiments that would affect food consumption and health. Our texts indicated, in fact, that the evolution of societies would bring about a degradation of moral values and of the environment. Through the centuries, man has pursued unfettered competition and today seeks ever more power and status. Nations are engaged in a frenetic arms race. The rich countries mobilize huge amounts of money for experimentation of all sorts. All these activities are aggravated by the development of the five scourges, which are desire/attachment, ignorance, pride, anger, and jealousy.

At the meeting in the Soviet Union, I proposed prescribing the precious pills *rine-chen rilbou* to treat the illnesses of their patients. I had some available, but clearly not in sufficient quantity. I was then taken to a hospital where I could observe men, women, and children contaminated by nuclear radiation. They asked me for a diagnosis. I took pulses, explained my findings. I was pleased that they were accepted by the other doctors who were present.

I had to leave Chernobyl to respond to an invitation to go to Mongolia, but I promised the doctors I would return as soon as my obligations there had been accomplished. I spent two days in the capital of Mongolia, then took a small plane to go to participate in the celebrations of the seven hundredth anniversary of the death of Genghis Khan. I discovered a country and traditions very close to our own. Stoupas were erected in many places, prayer flags fluttered in the wind. Just as with us, the Mongols counted the repetitions of the mantra with the help of their prayer beads. I visited hospitals here also, and I realized that these doctors were also using Tibetan medicine to treat their patients. They called the substances by names that seemed strange to me and I provided the Tibetan names. In a monastery, they showed me a very old statue of the Buddha, eighty *thangkas*, effigies of the protecting deities whose faces were highlighted in gold and decorated with coral, and a considerable number of texts. I was especially sensitive to the religious fervor of these people. At their urging, I led an expedition to collect plants in the neighboring mountains, but once we arrived, there were scarcely any to be found. I later returned to Mongolia to spend almost a year there.

Back in Chernobyl I visited more patients. Some that I had seen on my first visit had left the hospital but no-one explained why. Only thirteen patients to whom I had prescribed the precious pills were still there for me to question and examine. Their palpitations had disappeared; their eyebrows were beginning to grow back; their eye pain was less severe. Unfortunately, we could do no more than lessen their suffering. It was then that they made a proposal to me, which I welcomed with an evident interest and a little pride. It meant the full recognition of our medicine as evidenced by the construction of a hospital endowed with a Tibetan section. The officials of the department of health suggested that we return to Moscow to visit the regions where they thought it was possible to find the plants and substances necessary for fabricating our medicines. I returned to Dharamsala and 1990 (the year horse-iron) passed in negotiations and dealings with the Russians. During this time I trained some doctors in the process of purifying metals and others were prepared for research. I was rather optimistic about the preservation of our medical tradition, the one condition being the avail-ability of the materials.

I returned to Moscow in August 1991 (the year sheep-iron). Namguiel came with me. The project was taking shape and about twenty Tibetans could be appointed to this institute. All the documents were ready. We took a plane to the Mongolian capital along with nine Russians, then took another flight to the Chinese border. We spent about three weeks there looking for certain medicinal plants but we found very few, in any case they were insufficient for what we were planning to do. Disappointed, we returned to Moscow in September. The political events in the Soviet Union, lack of financial support, and especially lack of plants, finally prevented us from realizing the project. I left with a certain bitterness in my heart, but the essential, the recognition of the value of our medicine, had been accomplished.

Moscow, Paris, Rome, Zurich, Geneva, Mexico City, Tokyo, Lisbon, Sydney, Frankfurt, the great cities of the world were inviting me. They questioned me on the situation in Tibet, on life in the camps. Our medicine was and remains much appreciated by the Western world. At this time, I learned that the Chinese had spent ten thousand yuan on the restoration of Chothey. Circumstances were such that I was able to contribute a matching donation, which provoked an immediate reaction from the local authorities. But in reality, to reconstruct Chothey would require a considerable sum. I still feel a profound sadness about it today and wish so much that Chothey might live again.

It is 1996 (the year mouse-fire). I am seventy-four years old and I must now prepare myself to leave this body. I am convinced that I will never see Tibet again in this life. Since 1980, the year that I came to Dharamsala, I have done my best to help Men-Tsee-Khang to preserve our traditions. Four master-doctors now know the procedures for purification and detoxification of mercury and other metals. In the course of this year, thirteen practitioners have also benefited from instruction. Eighty students work under the permanent direction of professors. They are the future of our institution. In 1996 we have been able to prepare 109 kilos of mercury and several million pills. Foreigners have brought us help. Some have taught Western science to our students. Others have encouraged and helped us, and have offered us money, materials, and office staff. We now have microscopes and computers. Scientists throughout the entire world now know about and appreciate our work. But there remains much to do for Tibetan medicine to be recognized for its value and to find its true place, so that it may contribute to the well-being of humanity.

18

Epilogue: On the Threshold of the Great Voyage

To be born is already a step toward death. I often think about my own death, which nears. As a Buddhist, I consider it a natural process, a reality that I have admitted all along through my existence. No-one can escape it, and I see no reason to be disturbed about it. It is not a true end.

Every instant that I live brings me closer to that moment. I have prepared myself for it for a very long time, trying my best to apply the teachings of the Dharma. Living the last years of my life in proximity to His Holiness the fourteenth Dalai Lama, I have accepted even more strongly this evidence: only thoughts of love, compassion, goodness are essential. On this point, Tenzin Gyatso and Mahatma Gandhi deliver the same message, demanding of us that we love even our enemy. Since 1949 (the year cattle-earth) Communist China has occupied Tibet, imposing a pitiless policy of repression. However, though our enemy is cruel, sowing terror, violence and injustice, the Buddha tells us to love him. It must be understood that ignorance is at the source of all our sufferings and therefore of our behavior. It is only by dialogue that the Tibetan question will be resolved one day. This memoir bears witness so that the world will know that we Tibetans have suffered, and continue to suffer, under the Chinese boot. Beijing claims to have softened its policy of occupation. If one were to believe this, Tibetans may now practice their religion, pursue an education. Unfortunately, there is no truth to that. Oppressed in Tibet or free in exile, Tibetans do not accept the Chinese occupation; they endure it, physically and morally. Yet no occupying force will ever be able to vanquish the will and determination of the Tibetan people to survive, or undermine their confidence in the Dalai Lama, their spiritual and temporal guide.

Love and compassion play a primordial role in our existence. And tolerance. We should exert ourselves to lead a life directed by awareness of our actions. Thus, whatever happens, we will have nothing to regret.

At the age of seventy-seven, I keep my hope in the future. Throughout my life, I have tried my best to help others, friends and enemies alike. I have remained faithful to His Holiness the Dalai Lama. I will continue to serve him in the time that is left to me to live. Then one day I will leave. Perhaps I will be reborn as a simple monk at Chothey to help in the reconstruction of the monastery, or even a doctor at Men-Tsee-Khang to continue the work of my master, the Venerable Khenrab Norbu, or even . . .

May I work, if it should be needed,
To preserve always
The precious culture of the Dharma and of medicine,
For so long borne by the Tibetan tradition.

Appeal for Truth

You, Buddhas of the past, present and future, Bodhisattvas
   and Disciples,
Who have opened an ocean of limitless qualities,
Who consider every being as your only child,
Be attentive to this desperate petition
For the recognition of the Truth.

May the teachings of the Buddha which permit
the suppression of misery,
Spread well-being and prosperity throughout the world.
May the guardians of the Dharma of the doctrine
   and of the Dharma of realizations
Act to sustain the ten aspects of the practice.

In the grip of powerful evil actions,
Beings are ceaselessly borne off by pangs of affliction,
By all the fears, famine, weapons, and illness,
   so difficult to endure.
By your powers, may each of their breaths be like an ocean
   of peace and happiness.

Especially, may the guardians of the Dharma of the Land of
   Snows
Release the powerful forces of Compassion,
To quickly stop these tears and this blood
That armies of pitiless barbarians, come
   from a darkened country, have caused to flow.

These barbarians of infamous behavior, provoked
   by the perturbations of bad spirits,
These objects of compassion work to their own ruin
   and that of others.

May these gatherings of undisciplined beings obtain the
  eye of Wisdom,
And spread love and peace everywhere.

The sense of my wish, nurtured in the deepest part of my
  heart,
Is that purity and freedom regain all of Tibet,
May the celebration of harmonious coexistence of the
  spiritual and the temporal
Come to pass as soon as possible.

O Protectors, in your compassion, take care
of the Teaching and of its guardians, of the people
  and of their representatives,
Of those who have sacrificed their possessions and their
  lives and endured so much cruelty.

Under the eye of the Victorious One,
You, Chenrezik, Protector who watches over Tibet,
In keeping with our great prayer,
Let good fortune rain down soon.

From the interdependence of the profound reality of
  appearance and of the void,
From the strength of truthful words, from the power of
  compassion of the Three Excellent Jewels,
And from the power of the infallible truth of the law of
  causality,
May this prayer of truth be realized rapidly and without
  obstacle.

His Holiness Tenzin Gyatso,
Fourteenth Dalai Lama

Endnotes

1 This can also be a piece of wood.

2 In certain regions of Tibet, this ceremony takes place for a girl on the fourth day after the birth.

3 The Buddha explained that in order to attain perfection, one should develop compassion (a quality of the heart) and wisdom (a quality of intelligence) together. When the path has been entirely traversed, the practitioner becomes a Buddha or Enlightened One, which is to say a being who has awakened all the potentialities in him or herself and has brought them to their fullest flowering. The fundamental message of the Buddha is that all beings possess in themselves to the same extent the Buddha nature, which is the potentiality of becoming Buddha.

4 Milarepa (1040–1123): sage and poet who spent most of his life in grottos. His poems were not published in the West until 1962.

5 Situated in the State of Himachal Predesh (India), Dharamsala since 1960 has been the seat of the Tibetan government in exile and the place of residence of His Holiness the 14th Dalai Lama.

6 Chigatse, capital of the region of Tsang. In 1447 Guendune Droup (1391–1475), the first Dalai Lama, disciple of Je Tsongkhapa, founded the monastery of

Tachilhunpo, near Chigatse. Under the name of Guieloua Rinpoche [Precious Victor], he became the first abbot. Having established a printing press, Guendune Droup undertook the printing of *Kanguiour* and *Tenguiour* (the first is the collection of the Words of the Shakyamuni Buddha; the second the collection of commentaries composed later by Indian masters; these two collections are translations from Sanskrit into Tibetan). Tachilhunpo then became, by the decree of the fifth Dalai Lama, Ngawang Lobsang (1617–1682), the residence of the Panchen Lamas.

7 Seven varieties of garlic are used in Tibetan medicine. Nepalese merchants used to come at the time to look for these plants in Tibet and would resell them in their country, where they were used as condiments.

8 In Tibetan, *Dreulma*; feminine divinity of Buddhism, Tara is very popular in Tibet. She personifies the activity of all the Buddhas for the good of all living beings. She is also invoked as the liberator.

9 *Boumdrok* (in 13 volumes) and *Nyitri* (in 3 volumes) evoke vacuity in a more precise and detailed manner. Some families read the *Kadam* (a single volume), especially when they have been struck by misfortune, death, or malevolent spirits. One can also call upon the *Beunpo* for specific rituals especially aimed at repelling evil spirits. Once a year, after the harvest, villagers put together a certain amount of money and invite the monks to read the *Kanguiour*, which comprises a little more than one hundred volumes. The ceremonies last several days; fifty to sixty people help in the preparations for these very important celebrations, accomplishing profane tasks such as the preparation of the best possible foods.

10 Samadhiradjasoutra, *Ancient Futures: Learning from Ladakh*, Helena Norbert Hodge, London, Rider, 1991.

11 *Bodong*: Name of a place situated to the north-east of

Endnotes

Tachilhunpo. The complete name of the monastery is Nyemo Je Kar Chothey. The information obtained on the subject comes from a biography of Lotchen Bero, a scholar who lived at Chothey.

12 *Tulku*: The idea of reincarnation is integrated into the philosophical structure of Buddhism. A *tulku* is the reincarnation of a master from the past.

13 The Fifth Dalai Lama, Ngaouang Lobsang Gyatso (1617–1682), established the constitutional form of government that was maintained in Tibet until 1959. He also organized the temporal and spiritual hierarchies in the country. Such was his importance in the history of Tibet that he is known as the 'Great Fifth Dalai Lama'.

14 Tibetans also call him Kiabgoeun Rinpoche, 'Precious Protector'; Kiabgoeun Bouk, 'Internal Protector'; Lama Peunpo, 'Principal Lama', or simply Kundun, 'Presence'.

15 Amitabha enjoyed considerable popularity with the people in China, Japan and Tibet, and also in the Himalayas.

16 He reigned from 838 to 842. A great persecution took place at the same time in China (842–846). Langdarma was assassinated by a Tibetan monk, Pelki Dordje.

17 The 'historic' Buddha, who is at the origin of the Dharma, as it is still practiced today.

18 The monks would display all the *thangkas* on the festival of Kune Rik Dome Cheu, which usually begins on the twenty-second day of the twelfth month of the year and ends on the fifteenth day of the first month of the new year.

19 They say that it represented the terrifying aspect of Cheenrezik.

20 Sometimes the particle *la* is added as a mark of respect: *amchila*.

21 The first medical school, founded by the fifth Dalai Lama

at the monastery of Drepoung. It was eventually transferred to a monastic hospital-school complex called
Chagpori, the 'Mountain of Fire', on a hill of Lhasa, the
capital. Chagpori became the center of medicine in Tibet,
renowned in neighboring countries, especially Central
Asia, for the science dispensed by the lama-doctors. Once
established, Sanguie Gyatso, the regent of the fifth Dalai
Lama and doubtless the most powerful man in Tibet
at this time, decided that each monastery would house
a lama-physician trained at Chagpori. This was the beginning of 'public health' in Tibet.

22 In October 1913 a delegation left for Simla. An agreement
was signed 3 June, 1914, by Tibet, Great Britain and China,
marking the borders, a sensitive question for the Chinese
who wanted to affirm their full territorial sovereignty and
the authority of the government of the thirteenth Dalai
Lama, who wanted absolutely to observe the interests of
the populations of the Kham and the Amdo. Finally, in
refusing to sign, China did not recognize this document.

23 The birth name of the child, born at Taktser in the Amdo,
6 July, 1935, and recognized as the reincarnation of the
thirteenth Dalai Lama. Following the installation ceremonies, he assumed the name Tenzin Gyatso, fourteenth
Dalai Lama. The ceremony was fixed at 22 February, 1940,
by erudite astrological calculations.

24 He died in the year sheep-wood of the Tibetan calendar
(1955).

25 The sum represented then in Tibetan money five bills of
fifty *sang*. Tibet issued its own bills and postage stamps as
of 1912. They were printed by hand from wooden blocks
(xylographs) on paper made locally. The bills were printed
individually and the stamps in series of twelve. A great
variety of colors and printing qualities exist.

26 From the death of the thirteenth Dalai Lama and until his

successor assumed temporal power, Tibet was directed by two regents, Reting Rinpoche and Tagdra Rinpoche. The latter favored a conservative policy that seemed to be in total contradiction with the events that were shaking Tibet's neighboring countries. Nationalist China had aligned itself with the United States against Japan. That did not prevent it from maintaining annexationist views on the Roof of the World. Chang Kai-Chek had also sent to Lhasa one of his advisors, Sgen Tsung-lien, while the British asked Sir Basil Gould to represent them. The contacts did not proceed further.

27 The great masters Padma Sambhava and Je Tsongkhapa are considered incarnations of Manjushri the bodhisattva of transcendent wisdom. Padma Sambhava was born in the Udiyana in the north of India. He was a tantric master who contributed to the first introduction of Buddhism into Tibet and overcame forces hostile to it. He also helped in the construction of Samye, the first Tibetan Buddhist monastery. Je Tsongkhapa (1357–1419) was a great master of the tradition and founder of the *gelukpa* school in the tradition of the *kadam* school.

28 Ganden: one of the three principal *gelukpa* monasteries, along with Drepopung and Sera.

29 *Ganden Tripa*: title borne by the chief of the *gelukpa* line. *Ganden* is the name of the monastery, *tri* signifies throne in Tibetan. Literally, 'he who is titulary of the throne of Ganden'.

30 He studied in particular the *Gyushi* [the *Four Tantras*] and the *Baidurya Ngonpo* under the tutelage of Tekhang Jampa Thupuang, the *tulku* Jamyang Norbu, Drepung Khangsar Rinpoche, and Jamyang Khyentse, all of whom belonged to different orders of Tibetan Buddhism. Rongtsa Chachung Lobsang Damcheu Gyatso taught him about the foundations of the text *The White Lapis-lazuli*, and

about horoscopes and astrological calculations. From studying drawing, Khenrab Norbu better understood the *Rinchen-byung-gnas* lexicography. He also learned Sanskrit with the Mongolian *gueshe* Gadenpa, who based his teachings on the text *Brda-sprod-dbyangs-can-sgra-mdo*. Finally, Khenrab Norbu was taught philosophy by the lama Golok Jampel Reulpe Lodreu.

31 Among others: *Pegaeophyton*, *scapiflorum*, *Astragalus pastorius*, *Lagoti yumnanesis*, *Meconopsis horridula*, *Oxytropis subpoduoba*, *Saxifraga umbellulata*.

32 He would recite the *La me nel djor* and the *Guiu tok nying tik*.

33 The *Four Tantras*. Its complete title: *The Tantric Essence of Ambrosia: The Secret Oral Teaching of the Eight Branches of Medicine*. A summary of the *Four Tantras* is as follows: the *Root Tantra* touches on all illnesses and their examination; the *Tantra of Explanations* describes the doctrine of the therapy; the *Tantra of the Essential Instructions*, the most imposing of the four, gives all the details of the specific illnesses; and the *Final Tantra*. Together they are composed of 156 chapters, describing some 1,600 pathological states and no fewer than 2,993 medicinal substances.

34 Illnesses can be classed in different ways, but the most general is by disequilibriums of each of the three humors.

35 The uterus in a woman.

36 In the medicine mandala the Buddha holds a myrobolan tree in his hands.

37 Himalayan juniper, the berries of which, when burned like incense, have a curative effect on delirium caused by fever.

38 Just as the biliary calculus of elephants treats fever, bear bile cures liver problems, musk neutralizes septicemic infections and illnesses caused by worms.

39 This plant is a *tse-kam-nue-pa-ting-doe*. It is gathered only once when it is dry and its roots are still energetic. That is

where all the medicinal properties are concentrated. The *chou-tak* are used for gastritis, intestinal troubles, renal infections and serve as a stimulant. They are an ingredient in the preparation of antiseptic pills.

40 *Rang-nyi*, also known by the name of *tse-kam-nue-pa-ting-doe*. Its leaves and tubers are used for treating renal troubles and raising the body temperature.

41 This indication is useful only for Tibet. Because of the climate they only keep them a year in India.

42 The *rishis* are sages.

43 Moxibustion is a therapeutic method which consists of applying a heat source to the skin, either directly or at a slight distance.

44 In the Tibetan system the vertebrae are counted starting from the most prominent one at the base of the neck, which corresponds to the seventh cervical of the Western system. The sixth vertebra is considered the 'secret point of the life force'.

45 Honorific title given to the mother of the fourteenth Dalai Lama. Dekyi Tsering (1900–1981) was adored by the Tibetan people. In 1960 she sought refuge in India with His Holiness and she never saw her native country again. Later this same title was given to Jetsune Pema, younger sister of the Dalai Lama and President of the Tibetan Children's Village in Dharamsala. The National Assembly of the Tibetan people even designated Jetsune Pema as Mother of Tibet for her actions on behalf of the children in exile.

46 Inhabitants of the large eastern province of Kham, which was divided into two parts at the beginning of the twentieth century. The western part of Kham remained under the control of Lhasa; the eastern part was attached to Chinese Sechuan. The revolt of the Khampas affected both zones.

Glossary

Amala: term for mother.

Bardo: 'between', 'intermediate state'. Intermediate state between death and rebirth. At the moment of death, the being does not disappear completely. Leaving its physical body behind, its mental continuity passes through an intermediate stage before finding a new support for existence.

Beun: religious tradition active in Tibet before the introduction of Buddhism, and which persists today.

Bodhisattva: A person who has attained perfect enlightenment.

Buddhist schools: Tibetan Buddhism is of the *Mahayana* tradition, which spread in Tibet in the form of four schools: *Kaguiou*, *Nyingma*, *Sakya*, and *Gueloug*. These four schools still maintain their lines of transmission intact.

Chang: barley beer.

Chang-Sep-Char: residence of the Dalai Lama's family before the Chinese invasion, situated between the center of Lhasa and the Potala.

Chenrezik: the Buddha of Great Compassion; in Sanskrit, Avalokiteshvara. He is the protector of the country and its inhabitants. Much venerated in China under the name Guanyin, and in Japan under the name Kannon, where he is represented in a female form.

304

Glossary

Chupa: Tibetan dress worn by men and women.

Dalai Lama: *Dalai* is a Mongol word meaning 'ocean', and *Lama* is the Tibetan equivalent of the Indian term 'guru', which designates a spiritual master. Together, the two terms are often translated as 'Ocean of Wisdom'. But Dalai Lama is above all a title, that of the spiritual leader of Tibet, the most eminent religious figure recognized by the Buddhist world, who is also the temporal leader of Tibet and head of the government. The Dalai Lama is the human manifestation of Chenrezik, the Buddha of Great Compassion, considered the protector of the country. The title was first conferred on Seunam Gyatso (1543–1599) by the Mongol chief Altan Khan in 1578.

Dharma: this Sanskrit word can have several meanings, including the Buddha's teaching, the ultimate reality in the teachings, and the path to its attainment.

Dri: female yak.

Ganden Tripa: title given to the head of the *Gueloug* line. *Ganden* is the name of the *Gueloug* monastery, *tri* signifies 'throne', *pa* means 'person'. Literally, 'he who is the holder of the throne of Ganden'.

Gueshe: title of doctor of Buddhist philosophy awarded in the *Gueloug* school after difficult examinations.

Gyalyoum: honorific for the mother of the Dalai Lama. The honorific for the Dalai Lama's father is *gyeliap*.

Gyeltsap: regent designated by the *Kashag* to govern Tibet during the absence and the minorities of the Dalai Lamas.

Gyushi: the *Four Tantras*, texts containing the medical teachings.

Je Tsongkhapa: (1357–1419) founder of the *Gueloug* school, in continuity of the *kadam* tradition, of which he was the grand master.

Jokhang: principal temple of Lhasa, the Tibetan capital. The temple most venerated by Tibetan Buddhists, founded in the seventh century.

Joo: statue of the Shakyamuni Buddha, located in the heart of Jokhang. It is the most venerated in Tibet.

Kalachakra: divinity of tantric Tibetan Buddhism.

Karma: important concept of Buddhism. Etymologically, karma signifies action. Karmic law refers to the laws that govern actions and the results they incur.

Kashag: council of ministers, composed of three lay persons (the *kaleun*) and one religious [the *kaleun lama*], when Tibet was independent. Today the *Kashag*, reconstituted in exile, is composed of seven ministers (*kallums*).

Kata: white scarf, usually of silk, presented as a sign of greeting.

Kundun: one of the titles of the Dalai Lama.

Lhamenpa: on becoming personal physician of the Dalai Lama, an *amchi* is honored with this title, used today for any doctor of His Holiness.

Lossar: the new year. The ceremonies of the Tibetan new year begin on the twenty-ninth day of the twelfth month, the day of the *Goutor*, when all the negativities of the past year are exorcized. It is the occasion for numerous celebrations. The Tibetan calendar begins in the year 127 B.C. (2000=2127 of the Tibetan calendar.)

Mala: prayer beads used for counting mantras, similar to a rosary.

Mandala: ritual design used in Buddhism as in Hinduism as a support for meditation. The sand mandala is made of five different colors representing the five aggregates: form, feeling, recognition, composition, and consciousness.

Mani stone: stone engraved with the mantra *Om Mani Padme Hum*. Some are colored and can be large rocks; small ones may be piled up to form walls called *mendong*. They are found everywhere, in sacred places, near monasteries, and in villages.

Mola: term for grandmother.

Momo: traditional feast dish, resembling ravioli, filled with vegetables or meat.

Monlam: collective rituals of good wishes given at the new year.

Monlam Chenmo: literally, the 'Great Prayer'. Instituted by Je Tsongkhapa in 1409, this religious festival celebrated during the first fifteen days following the new year used to gather as many as fifty thousand people in Lhasa.

Moxibustion: therapeutic method consisting of applying heat sources to the skin.

Netchoung, oracle of: designates the person whose function it is to execute special ceremonies, during which he is penetrated by the spirit of a deity while he is in a trance; in this state, he delivers predictions. The Tibetans call this person *Kouten*, which signifies literally the 'physical support'. It is said that the spirit of *Netchoung* entered the body of a human for the first time in 1544. Thus, Drag Trang-gowa Lobsang Pelden became the first *Netchoung Kouten*.

Om Mani Padme Hum: the best-known mantra in Tibet; it is the mantra of Chenrezik, the Buddha of great Com- passion, who is considered the protector of the country. The six syllables of the mantra symbolize the six realms of existence and are translated as 'Hail to the Jewel in the Lotus'. This mantra is the essence of all Buddhist mantras and prayers.

Padma Sambhava: Tantric master, born in the Udiyana, in the north of India, who contributed to the first introduction of Buddhism in Tibet by subduing forces that were hostile to it. He also helped in the construction of Samye, the first Tibetan Buddhist monastery.

Pala: term for father.

Poudja: religious ceremony.

Ramotche Tsouklakhang: one of the most venerated temples of Tibetan Buddhism, situated in Lhasa.

Regent: person who directs the country in the absence of the Dalai Lama or during his minority.

Reincarnation: see *tulku*.

Rinpoche: honorific designating a spiritual master who is qualified and recognized. Example: Dalai Lama is a Mongol name used also by the Chinese and Westerners. The Tibetans call him Gyalwa Rinpoche: the Precious Victor.

Samsara: cycles of existence.

Sang: Tibetan currency.

Sangha: a Sanskrit word meaning 'lot', a group of like-minded people, a cohesive community.

Soutra: the *soutras* are the texts containing the original teachings of the Buddha.

Tachi delek: a term of greeting for all occasions. It means 'good luck'.

Tantra: the tantras are the teachings and the writings that establish the foundation of Vajrayana.

Tashilhunpo: monastery founded by Guendune Droup, the first Dalai Lama, disciple of Tsongkhapa, in 1447 near Chigatse.

Thamzing: meaning literally 'to fight', session of public criticism applied by the Communist Chinese; the person under examination stands for several hours facing a group assembled for the session. The person's family, children, friends can be obliged to participate in criticizing, humiliating and beating the victim, who often reaches the point of wishing for or requesting a quick death.

Thangka: Tibetan painting based on the Indian religious art of the Pala dynasty. In the tradition of the Indian Buddhist teachings, the Tibetans have scrupulously followed the instructions of the Nepalese Buddhists. *Thangka* painting developed in central Tibet in the seventh century under the reign of King Songtsen Gampo.

Tsampa: toasted barley flour.

Tsokrampa: *Gueshe* (see above) of the second order. The examination is given in Lhasa during the festival of Tsok-Cheu Monlam.

Tsotru: the precious pill having purified mercury as its base.

Tulku: a *tulku* is the reincarnation of a past master. The idea of reincarnation is integral to the philosophical structure of Buddhism.

Bibliography

Avedon, John F., *Loin du Pays des Neiges*, Calmann-Lévy.

Barraux, Roland, *Histoire des Dalaï-Lamas*, Paris, Albin Michel, 1993.

Bell, Charles, *The Land of the Lamas*, London, Secley Services and Co, 1929.

- *The Religion of Tibet*, Oxford, Oxford University Press, reissued 1968

- *Portrait of a Dalaï-Lama*, London, Wisdom Publications, reissued 1987.

- *Tibet Past and Present*, Delhi, Motilal Banarsidass, reissued 1992.

Clifford, Terry, *La Médecine tibétaine bouddhique et sa psychiatrie*, Paris, Dervy-Livres, 1991.

Collectif, *Tibet, des journalistes témoignent*, Paris, L'Harmattan, 1992.

- *Tibet, l'envers du décor*, Geneva, Olizane, 1993.

- *Tibet, la solution l'indépendance*, Geneva, Olizane, 1995.

Comité juridique d'enquête sur la question du Tibet, *Le Tibet et la République populaire de Chine*, Geneva, Commission internationale de juristes, 1997.

Commission internationale de juristes, *La Question du Tibet et la Primauté de droit*, Geneva, 1960.

Bibliography

Das, Sarat Chandra, 'The Hierarchy of the Dalaï-Lamas', *Journal of the Asiatic Society of Bengal*, 1904.

- *Tibetan Studies*, Calcutta, K. P. Bagghi & Co., 1984.
- *Lhassa and Central Tibet*, Delhi, W. W. Rockhill, reissued 1988.

Deshayes, Laurent, *Histoire du Tibet*, Paris, Fayard, 1997.

Djamyang, Norbou, *Un Cavalier dans la neige*, Paris, Maisonneuve, 1981.

Donnet, P. A., *Tibet mort ou vif*, Paris, Gallimard, 1990.

Eco-Tibet France, *Tibet, Environnement et développement*, Savoie, Editions Prajna, 1993.

Fromaget, A., *Océan du pure mélodie*, Vie et chants du sixième Dalaï-Lama, Paris, Dervy, 1995.

Goldstein, Melvyn C., *A History of Modern Tibet*, University of California Press, 1986.

Harrer, Heinrich, *Sept Ans d'aventures au Tibet*, Paris, Arthaud, 1983.

Lamothe, M.-J. *Les Cent Mille Chants de Milarépa*, Paris, Fayard, 3 vol., 1988.

- *La Vie de Milarépa*, Paris, Seuil, 1997.
- *Sur les pas de Milarépa*, Paris, Albin Michel, 1998.

Lillico, S., 'The Panchen-Lama', Shangaï, *The China Journal*, vol. XXI, 1934, pp. 96–9.

Malik, Inder L. *Dalaï-Lama of Tibet*, New Delhi, Uppal Publishing House, 1984.

Maraini, Fosco, *Tibet Secret*, Paris, Arthaud, 1990.

Martynov, A. S., *On the Status of the Fifth Dalaï-Lama*.

Mehra, *Tibetan Policy (1904–1937), Conflict between the 13th Dalaï-Lama and the 9th Panchen*, Leyde, ed. J. Brill, 1976.

Mullin, Glenn H., *Selected Works of the Dalaï-Lama III, Essence of Refined Gold*, Ithaca, Snow Lion, reissued 1982.

- *Selected Works of the Dalaï-Lama VII*, Ithaca, Snow Lion, reissued 1985.

- *Selected Works of the Dalaï-Lama II, Tantric Yogas of Sister Niguma*, Ithaca, Snow Lion, reissued 1985.
- *Path of the Bodhisattva Warrior, The Life and Teachings of the Thirteenth Dalaï-Lama*, Ithaca, Snow Lion, 1988.
- *Mystical Verses of a Mad Dalaï-Lama*, Weaton, First Quest Edition, 1994.

Ngapo, Ngawang Jigme, *Tibet*, PML Editions, 1989.

Patt, D., *A Strange Liberation, Tibetan Lives in Chinese Hands*, Ithaca, Snow Lion, 1992.

Példèn, Guiatso, *Le Feu sous la neige*, Arles, Actes Sud, 1997.

Pemajetsun, *Tibet, mon histoire*, propos recueillis par Gilles Van Grasdorff, Paris, Ramsay, 1996.

Richardson, H. E., *Tibet and its History*, Oxford University Press, 1962.
- *A Short History of Tibet*, New York, Dutton and Co., 1962.
- 'The Dalaï-Lamas', London, *Occasional Paper of the Institute of Tibetan Studies*, no. 1, Shambala, Pandect Press Ltd, 1971, pp. 19–30.

Rinchen, Dolma Taring, *Daughter of Tibet*, London, 1970.

Rockhill, Woodwille W., *The Dalaï-Lamas of Lhasa and their Relationships with the Manchu Emperors of China, 1644–1908*, Leyde, 1910.

Samten, Gyaltsen Karmay and Heather, Stoddard, *Secret Vision of the Fifth Dalaï-Lama*, Serindia, 1988.

Shakabpa, W. D., *Tibet, a Political History*, New York, Potala Publications, 1984.

Snellgrove, D. L. and Richardson, H., *A Cultural History of Tibet*, London Weidenfeld and Nicolson, 1968.

Sogyal, Rinpotché, *Le Livre tibétain de la Vie et de la Mort*, Paris, La Table ronde, 1993.

Stein, R. A., *La Civilisation tibétaine*, Paris, L'Asiathèque-Le Sycomore, reissued 1981.

Bibliography

Subba, T. B., *Flight and Adaptation, Tibetan refugees in the Darjeeling Sikkim Himalaya*, Dharamsala, LTWA, 1990.

Surkhang, Wangchen Gélek, 'The Critical Years: The Thirteenth Dalaï-Lama', in *Tibet Journal*.

Tibetan Young Buddhist Association, *Tibet, the Facts*, Dharamsala, TYBA, reissued 1990.

Tokan, Tada, *The Thirteenth Dalaï-Lama*, Tokyo, 1965.

Van Walt van Praag, Michael, *The Status of Tibet*, Colorado, 1987.

Wang, Furen et Suo, Wenqing, *Highlights of Tibetan History*, Beijing, New World Press, 1984.

Winnington, Alan, *Tibet*, London, 1957.

Wu, Harry, *Retour au Laogai*, Paris, Belfond, 1996.

Ya, Hanzhang, *The Biographies of the Dalaï-Lamas*, Beijing, Foreign Languages Press, 1991.

Younghusband, Francis, *India and Tibet*, 1905.

His Holiness the Fourteenth Dalaï-Lama, *Universal Responsibility and the Good Heart*, Library of Tibetan Works and Archives, 1980.

- *Four Essential Buddhist Commentaries*, Library of Tibetan Works and Archives, 1980.

- *Kindness, Clarity and Insight*, New York, Snow Lion, 1984.

- *Mon pays et mon peuple*, Geneva, Olizane, 1984.

- *Opening the Mind and Generating a Good Heart*, Library of Tibetan Works and Archives, 1985.

- *Au loin la Liberté*, Paris, Fayard, 1990.

- *Enseignements essentiels*, Paris, Albin Michel, 1984.

- *Comme en éclair déchire la nuit*, Paris, Albin Michel, 1992.

- *Cent éléphants sur un brin d'herbe*, Paris, Le Seuil, 1991.

- *La Méditation au quotidien*, Geneva, Olizane, 1992.

- *Terre des Dieux, malheur des hommes*, entretien avec Gilles Van Grasdorff, Paris, Lattès, 1994.
- *Dialogues on Universal Responsibility and Education*, Library of Tibetan Works and Archives, 1995.
- *The Power of Compassion*, HarperCollins India, 1995.

And numerous Tibetan texts consulted in Dharamsala.

Tibet: Geography and Demographics

Size: 2.5 million square kilometers.

Capital: Lhasa.

Population: 6 million Tibetans. 8 million Chinese.

Religion: 90 per cent Buddhist (*beun* tradition, indigenous to Tibet); Islam and Catholicism are also practiced.

Language: Tibetan (Tibetan-Burman language family). Chinese is the official imposed language.

Common food/drink: *Tsampa* (toasted barley flour); salted buttered tea.

Average altitude: 4,000 meters.

Highest mountain: Chomo Langma (Mount Everest), 8,848 meters.

Fauna: Yak, bharal (blue sheep), musk deer, Tibetan antelope, gazelle, kiang (wild donkey), panda, and ibex.

Birds: Crane (black-necked), lammergeier, large crested grebe, bald goose, iridescent duck, ibis.

Major ecological aspects: Massive deforestation in the eastern part of Tibet, poaching of large mammals; excessive exploitation of minerals and other natural resources.

Average rainfall: Varies greatly. In the west, from 1mm in January to 25mm in July. In the east, from 25–50mm in January to 800mm in July.

Mineral resources: Bauxite, uranium, iron, copper, chromium, carbon, salt, mica, lithium, tin, gold and petrol.

Principal rivers: Zachu (Mekong), Dritchou (Yangtse), Matchou (Huangho), Gyelmo Ngoultchou (Salween), Tsangpo (Brahmapoutre), Senge Khabab (Indus), and Langchen Khabab (Sutlej).

Economy: Tibetans: essentially agricultural and domestic animal breeding. Chinese: government, commerce and services.

Provinces: U-Tsang (central Tibet), Amdo (north-eastern Tibet), Kham (south-eastern Tibet), Ngari (south-western Tibet), Chang Tang (northern Tibet).

Neighboring countries: India, Nepal, Bhutan, Burma (Myanmar), Eastern Turkestan, Mongolia and China.

Flag: A mountain, snow leopards, a sun with red and blue rays. Illegal in Tibet.

Chief of state: His Holiness the Fourteenth Dalai Lama (complete title: Jetsune Ngaouang Lobsang Yeche Tenzin Gyatso Sisoum Ouanguiour Tsounpa Mepe De Pelsangpo).

Government in exile: Democratic (parliamentary rule: 46 deputies elected every five years).

Government in Tibet: Communist.

Relations with China: Colonial.

Status: Occupied country.

Acknowledgements

I especially thank:

The translators from Tibet into English who assisted Dr Choedrak and Gilles Van Grasdorff in Dharamsala.

For the simultaneous translation: Kesang Yangzom, Tenzin Rabgyal for their continuous help, their talent and their support for the accomplishment of this project.

For the written translation: first, Phunestok, and his assistant Khedup Woeser, for their remarkable work, their patience and their kindness. And Dr Namgyal Tenzin for the quality of his translations of all the texts dealing with medicine.

For the research on Khenrab Norbu: the material was gathered in collaboration with Sonam Rinchen and Ngawang Soepa.

In France, thanks to Geraldine Le Roy for the enormous work of translating the 67 cassettes and other documents from English into French, in total more than 2,000 pages. Besides her talent, she brought her support and her faith in this project.

Jean Lassale and Jacques Krischer for their continued support.

The Office of Tibet and Wangpo Bashi for their collaboration.

Ngaouang Dakpa for his careful reading of the text, and thanks, also, to all his family.

This work would not have been possible without the especially warm welcome of the Tibetan government in exile and the entire Tibetan community.

My thanks go first to Dawa Thondup, former representative of His Holiness in France, who helped me establish contact with Dr Tenzin Choedrak, and warned me about the many risks I was going to encounter. Thanks also to Madame Kunzang D. Yuthok, present representative of His Holiness in Paris.

In Dharamsala, my thanks go particularly to Tempa Tsering, Secretary of the Department of Information and International Relations, for his confidence and his friendship, and to the entire Tibetan government in exile; To Jetsune Pema who organized everything at the Cottage, the site of so many meetings; to Pelden Gyatso, my friend; to the Oracle of Netchoung. In France, to Dagpo Rinpoche, for his unfailing support.

I especially wish to thank Gilbert Buesco, Professor of Tibetan at the Guepele Institute, author of *Parlons Tibetans* (Harmattan, 1988), for his contributions on the questions about the Dharma, Tibetan medicine, and the phonetic transcription of the Tibetan words. (Institut Guepele – Tibetan Institute – founded by Dagpo Rinpoche, Chemin de la Passerelle, 77250 Veneux-les-Sablons, France.)

And finally, my thanks to Claude Huriet, president of the *Association des amitiés parlementaires pour le Tibet au Senat*, Louis de Broissia and Jean-Jacques Robert; my friendship also to Leon Zeches and his family; to Andre

Acknowledgements

Heiderscheid; to Olivier Masseret; to Sofia and to Khoa; to Anne-Marie and Madame Gilbert Collard, our shared friendship; and to Marie . . .

G.V.G.

You may make a contribution to Men-Tsee-Khang or to the reconstruction of the Chothey monastery by contacting directly:

Dr Tenzin Choedrak
Men-Tsee-Khang
Tibetan Medical and Astrological Institute of
    His Holiness the Dalai Lama
Gangchen Kyishong
Dharamsala – 176215 (HP) India

If you wish to sponsor Tibetan religious or lay persons who are in difficulty, you may contact:

The Office of Tibet
1 Culworth Street
London NW8 7AF
UK
Tel: 44-20-7722-5378
Fax: 44-20-7722-0362
E-mail: info@tibet.com